Parenting
with Values

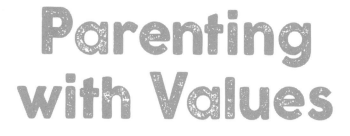

Parenting with Values

12 Essential Qualities
Your Children Need
and How to Teach Them

Christiane Kutik

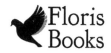

Floris
Books

Translated by Matthew Barton

First published in German as *Herzensbildung: Von der Kraft der*
Werte im Alltag mit Kindern by Verlag Freies Geistesleben in 2016
First published in English by Floris Books in 2018

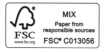

 Also available as an eBook

British Library CIP data available
ISBN 978-178250-482-5
Printed in Printed in Great Britain
by TJ International

Contents

Foreword

In our modern world of myriad possibilities, there is much to be thankful for: plentiful food, advanced technology and excellent healthcare, to name but a few. For our children, the world is at their fingertips: there are hundreds of TV channels, the entire internet to explore, and countless forms of entertainment. These things certainly keep children occupied and we might tell ourselves that they are lucky to have so many advantages. Yet this fast-paced modern world has its downsides too, and it is easy to become overwhelmed by the demands of our busy lives and lose sight of what is really important to ourselves and to our children. Take a step back, for a moment, and ask: what kind of parents do we really want to be, and what do our children really need from us?

There are things that will always be important to children, whether they realise it or not. Children will always want to feel secure: to know that they are valued and have a place in the world. Children will always appreciate independence: being encouraged to do things for themselves and joyfully finding out that they can. Children will always love it when their parents do nurturing things with them: when they take the time to listen to them or to explore the world's small miracles together.

Above all, children need warm-hearted attentiveness from us. They need us to show them the values by which they will best live their lives: self-respect, truthfulness and a real interest in the world. It is this sense of being fully present, of living a full life and of leading by example that is really important to raising our children – not giving them lots of material things that might entertain them for a little while but ultimately leave them unfulfilled.

The challenge for us as parents while bringing up our children is to break away from the busy modern world, engage our hearts and embrace what is truly important in life. I believe there are fundamental values that all children need, and we can give these to them simply by living those values every day ourselves.

My hope is that this book will inspire you to embrace parenting with values and show how, through small actions, we can enliven and enthuse our children and help them spread their wings. Try living these values, and watch the young eyes in your household shine with humour and delight.

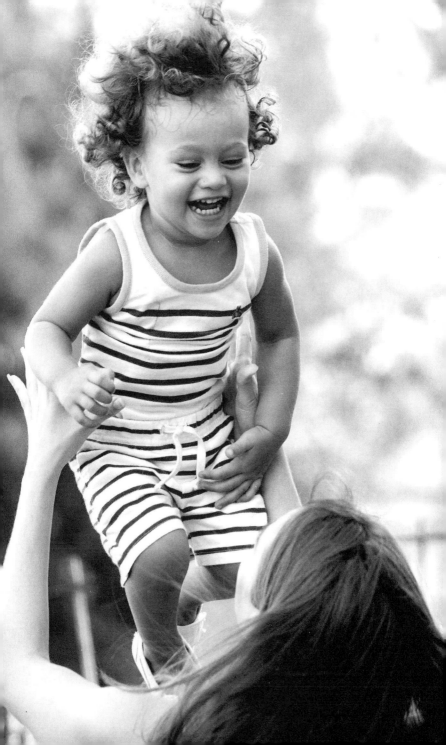

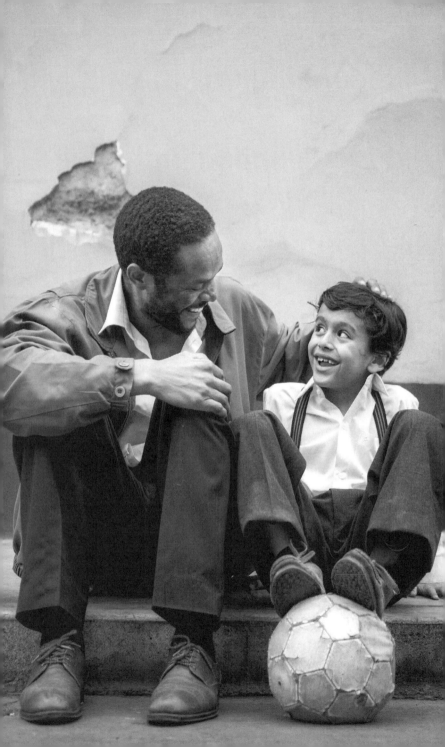

Introduction:
Helping the Heart to Grow

A six-year-old boy sitting next to his father suddenly asks him out of the blue, 'There are more good people than bad people, aren't there, Dad?'

His father looks thoughtful for a moment, then replies warmly, 'Yes, there are. And do you know, every day moments come when you and I can make life better!'

In current-day parenting, we can find ourselves focusing on behaviours we want or don't want from our children, and skills we think they need to develop. Considering 'values' might seem a little out of step with the modern world. Yet family life and our relationships with children are necessarily heavily laden with our values, for good or ill. As parents and caregivers, we are always demonstrating ways of being in the world with others and within ourselves. We are helping children to grow as emotional and moral beings. So I would encourage thinking about what might seem an old-fashioned idea: the development of character. Our children's wellbeing is dependent on the growth and learning not just of body and mind, but also of the heart.

We can all take small actions every day to make life kinder and richer, starting with considering how we ourselves behave towards, and how we communicate with, our children. Commands like, 'Don't tell lies!', 'Eat nicely!' and 'Don't swear!' are certainly direct, but they are usually less effective than modelling good behaviour for children ourselves. We can make sure *we* speak truthfully. We can show *our* good manners. We can make sure *we* don't swear.

We can all try to take more care. None of us is perfect, but we can take notice of our own faults and try to remedy them. This is an important example to set for children: that character, and our hearts, can develop if we take care of them.

It might be uncomfortable to witness our children reflecting our flaws back at us, but we can certainly learn from the experience. As Goethe said, 'A growing person will always be grateful.'[1] Remember, as parents we are still growing too, and we learn a great deal when we closely observe the natural, warm-hearted impulses children bring with them into the world.

Heart to heart

Take a moment to notice how much little children love sharing. All infants, to begin with, have this wonderful quality. But we adults can often unintentionally hinder it. Does this scene sound familiar?

> A father hands his daughter a piece of apple. The little girl takes it, bites off a piece, then offers the rest back to her father so he can have a bite too.
> But rather than sharing, he is frustrated. 'No,' he says. 'Eat up!'

It is natural to want our children to be nourished and to eat the food we give them; indeed, in every way, we want them to have what they need. Giving our children things that are 'just for you' might seem like the best way to parent – and the best way to please them. But what we see as generosity and nurturing can suppress children's natural warmth of heart.

The little girl who wanted her father to have a piece of apple might keep trying for a while to offer things she has, but if she is only ever rebuffed eventually she will assume her gifts are not wanted and she will stop. Yet children long to be taken seriously by grown-ups. How much better would it be to accept the gift given with such generosity of spirit and to encourage this impulse in our children?

Smiling is infectious

Children reflect genuine, vivid joyfulness when we really *see* them, when they sense our warm smile, for no particular reason, shining upon them. Smiling makes an immediate connection between people and warms our hearts – and that's what the world needs. Smiling is infectious: when we give, it comes straight back.

A smile is enough

Over one hundred studies have shown that rewarding children's values by giving them material things will 'weaken internal motivation'.[2] One of these studies, with two groups of infants aged twenty months, involved the adult participant clearing her desk and dropping a pencil. In the first group, the children who picked it up and gave it back to her were each given a small reward, while in the second they received a friendly smile. The researchers found that children rewarded materially soon lost the spontaneous urge to help, the children who received a smile did not. The smile affirmed the relationship the children were trying to build.

Nowadays, there are so many toys and technologies that can give children fleeting pleasure, and it is natural for us to want our children to have whatever they desire. However, the risks of using these as rewards for natural impulses should be heeded. Let's cherish our children's innate capacity for generosity and loving assistance, rather than feeling we need to reward them for it with more than love and smiles.

A warm greeting

Every encounter with our children has the potential for joy. This is why greeting them first thing in the morning is so important. Share a hug and say their name. Showing that we are happy to see our children gets the day started on a hopeful footing, and it only takes a couple of seconds. The same is true of giving a warm farewell when it is time to go to school or to nursery. These small gestures strengthen our children emotionally and make them feel loved.

Building emotional resilience

Helping our children to grow morally and emotionally is integral to our role as parents. However much we might wish otherwise, there are many negative influences around them. We might not be able to change the world, but we can help our children to build emotional resilience and give them the tools they need to thrive.

As parents, we can stand up for our values and beliefs. We can show our children what good, caring behaviour looks like and watch them bring those qualities into their own lives. This will bequeath our children a firm place in the world and comfort in their own being. Have courage: parenting with values will strengthen you and your child immeasurably.

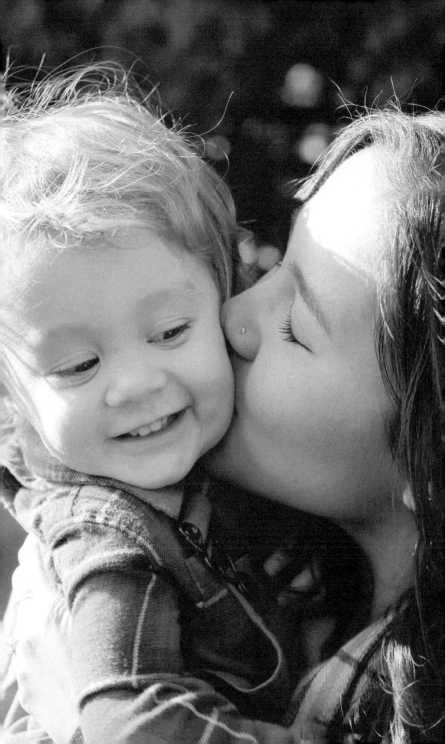

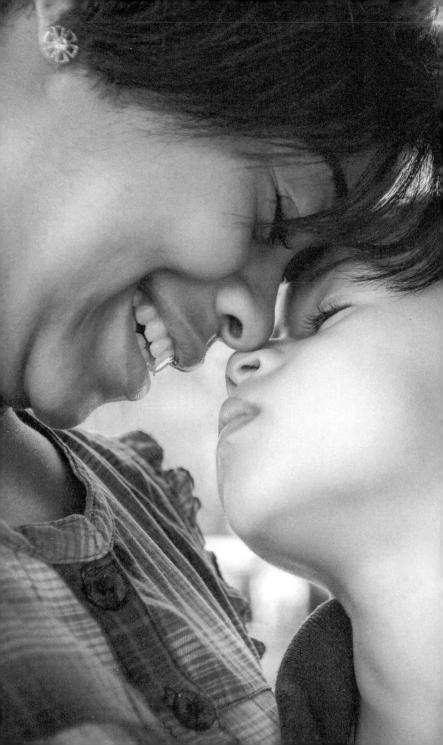

Security

Comforting and calming

A small boy falls over. His mother reaches for her bag and calls, 'Wait a moment, where are the Arnica pills?'

Another mother says: 'Look here are some – I always carry them with me.'

The boy's mother gives him the pills and asks a lot of questions: 'Where does it hurt? Is it bad? Come on, tell me darling!'

The sobbing child refuses to be comforted.

Compare that imagined scene with this one:

A small boy falls over. His mother picks him up, holds him, strokes his back. She sings quietly:

Three days of falling rain
Then the sun comes out again
And all will be well.

When I visualise this second scene, it is easy for me to imagine a child who is bumped but not badly hurt getting up from his mother's lap soon afterwards and skipping off, comforted, the pain of the bump seemingly soothed. Children often calm down quite quickly when we hold them and sing to them – in other words, when they feel closeness and safety.

Security is a basic human need

Our need for security goes far beyond bumps on the knee and momentary comforting. One of the mothers I talked with when I was thinking about this book told me how aware she was that her daughter didn't need most things that money could buy – expensive clothing and toys or big outings – rather she needed 'a familiar, trusted, warm adult who is always there for her'.

Children are very much dependent on a benevolent Other who shows interest in them and gives them a sense of safety and security. This brings the feeling of being in the right place – of being 'right' altogether.

Children need 'nest warmth'. They want to be accepted, to know: 'This is where I belong, and this is where I get support and help.'

Children want to be loved

Children want to feel they are loved just as they are and because of who they are. They need their parents to like them, and to show them they like them.

As parents, we can choose to show our children we like them as they are, rather than feeling we must always be urging them to change somehow: not to be so shy, to have more friends, to be more focused, more diligent, different.

Children thrive when they can blossom, when they aren't constrained by having to live up to other people's strong desires and feelings. Child psychologist Alice Miller talks about the importance of children feeling they can express their own self and their own feelings, perhaps especially the negative feelings. It is harmful to small children if they consistently feel they must be cheerful for the sake of others – that they cannot be sad or afraid or angry because others' needs come first.[3]

No time?

In the busy rush of modern life, it gets harder to give children a sense of security. Many parents are pressured with financial commitments, long office hours and daily stress. Many would love to spend more time with their children.

But then when they do have time to be with their children, parents are often physically present, but not fully available. Even babies can feel when others are distracted. Unsatisfied, they will keep demanding their parents' attention.

Imagine a two year old on his balance bike.

He wants to show his mother a new trick.

'Look Mummy!' he calls out happily, and lifts his feet up high as he rides.

But his mum is busy answering a message on her phone.

'Mummy, look!' The child tries again.

'Yes, I'm looking,' she calls back. She glances up and then returns to her phone screen.

'Mummy, why aren't you looking?'

'But I'm here,' she replies.

Being physically present isn't enough for children

Being physically present but mentally absent won't satisfy children's need for security. They need their parents' minds to turn to them. Children who sense that a device is more important than they are cannot feel secure.

Imagine how it feels inside when you at last get an outing with a parent you love, only for the parent to be constantly sending messages to other people.

Note, too, that babies can go for a long walk with their parent without being aware the parent is there, for example if the buggy faces forward and the parent is listening to headphones and never speaks to them.

What about cuddling in front of the TV?

Watching TV is something you can do together, but, again, it is distracted, so it won't give children a full sense of security.

The father of a five year old argued with me on this.

'We always watch together,' he said. 'She sits on my lap and I hold her.' He added, 'Sometimes it seems to me that cuddling is more important to her than the programme.'

'If that's the case,' I asked him, 'why do you bother turning the TV on at all?'

He pondered that. Eventually he said, 'You're right, I suppose... It's just a habit. I'll try not having it on. I want to have real time with my daughter.'

There are better ways of being close to children than sitting together in front of a screen. Indeed some psychologists believe screens are harmful for babies and young children (see, for example, Manfred Spitzer, who researches brain development).[4]

We are most in touch with children when...

...we engage personally and directly with them and talk with them. Often caregivers hold back from talking with their babies and small children because they believe little ones can't understand them, so what is the point? But even in earliest infancy, babies are completely receptive to heartfelt contact, to a friendly face, to someone who smiles and nods at them. Smile at a child in a shopping queue or at the bus stop and see how their eyes open wide, how they start to smile back: how pleased they are. Then recognise how much more important it is that loved caregivers do this, given children's reliance on direct contact with their parents and carers.

Consciously nurturing connection

We all have other things to do besides being with children, and yet children are more important than any task or message. Do show your children you know this: when you have time together try to avoid distractions and interruptions. Look and smile at your child, and chat with them. You'll be rewarded with their shining eyes the moment they feel your real attention.

As well as consciously giving our full attention to children, there are many little rituals we can cultivate in daily life to help nurture security.

Greeting and taking leave are vital

Greeting children and taking leave of them attentively and lovingly are some of the most important tools we have for acknowledging them and fostering a sense of security. Be mindful of this, not just in the morning and evening, but also during the day. Give eye contact, a touch, a kiss or a few warm words.

Sadly, parents often make do with a cursory 'Hello' or go without greetings entirely, and tell me that their children don't like affectionate gestures and words. But I would urge all parents and carers to persist in the attempt. Persevere with your affection: show your children that even if they are growing older they are too precious for you to simply pass by as you arrive or leave.

A father of teenagers told me: 'In our family we have always greeted one another with warmth and I think it has had an impact on our children. People often think ours are especially easy children, that they rarely challenge us. But I wonder whether they are copying what we've modelled for them: they are treating us as we treat them.'

Warmth and respect are wonderful qualities to learn at home, and they flow from a deep sense of security.

One of the mothers attending a parenting course of mine decided to give her fourteen-year-old daughter a special greeting one morning. 'It's so lovely that you exist!' she said, looking at her and giving her a hug.

Surprised, her daughter replied, 'Did you learn that at your course yesterday, Mum?'

'We both had to laugh,' the mother reported. 'But then we ate breakfast together and for the first time in months we really talked properly.'

Keeping in contact

Children long to be in real contact with people, especially with people they love. We cannot always be with them so we don't know what they have confronted in a day – bullying? Small humiliations and unfairness? Disappointments? Pressure from other children to do things that aren't comfortable? Disturbing images and stories? We can make all the difference if we are close enough to notice when our children are anxious or troubled. Children need parents who stand by them, and not only say 'You can tell me everything' but really mean it too. They need parents who stay in close contact.

How to listen when you think there's a problem

Lea is nine years old. Her mother noticed that she hasn't been herself recently. 'What's wrong?' her mother asked. 'Is anything wrong at school?'

Lea looked down at the floor.

'With the other children?'

She shook her head.

'Come on, tell me!' her mother urged. But because her daughter didn't volunteer an immediate answer, she turned away, saying, 'OK, if nothing's wrong...'

Later, in a parenting workshop with me, she complained that her daughter wouldn't tell her anything. Other parents confirmed they have the same experience with their children.

Children are not an information bureau. But when troubled, they do want to talk. Before they can open up, though, they need to be quite sure that Mum or Dad is really inwardly receptive, that they are genuinely willing to listen. In the workshop, we discussed how we can show we are open to hearing feelings.

The next time Lea's mother noticed her nine year old worrying about something, she said, 'Come on, let's go for a little walk together.'

At first Lea didn't want to. But in the end she came along.

Outside, walking side by side, it was easier to talk – especially because Lea's mother remembered the discussion at the workshop and was careful not to pressure or probe her child.

Instead, after walking together for a while, she related a difficult situation she herself experienced as a child. And then she fell silent but stayed inwardly receptive, and carried on walking with her daughter.

Suddenly Lea started to speak.

It often takes time for children to open up. They only do so if they feel that the adult they are with is really willing to engage, and won't just offer a pat answer for everything.

Giving time and being willing to engage is the way to nurture security.

And then sometimes the opening up can happen very spontaneously – perhaps at the weekend after a cushion fight in the parents' bed, with much laughter and no losers.

And boundaries are important too

Giving security requires a listening, open presence. But it doesn't mean living without boundaries, or giving limitless attention to every grievance and upset. When children overstep the mark, it remains our role to show them where the limits lie instead of mollycoddling them. Otherwise they learn to think of themselves as the centre of the universe around which everything else should revolve. Similarly, if we clear every stone from their path they never learn to endure frustration or rivalry.

Child psychoanalyst Judith Jackson says it is important for children to learn they are not the sole focus of the family.[5] In households where one parent is with the children more than another, it can be a valuable role for the less-involved parent (often still the father) to notice and mention when they see children are failing to listen, or are taking advantage of the at-home parent and crossing boundaries.

Giving children security means following a middle path, listening, yet never simply governed by the children's wishes. We need to watch that in our responses we are not motivated solely by seeking our children's love – for children love their parents anyway, even if this isn't always apparent.

To be able to give security we must also keep seeking our own equilibrium.

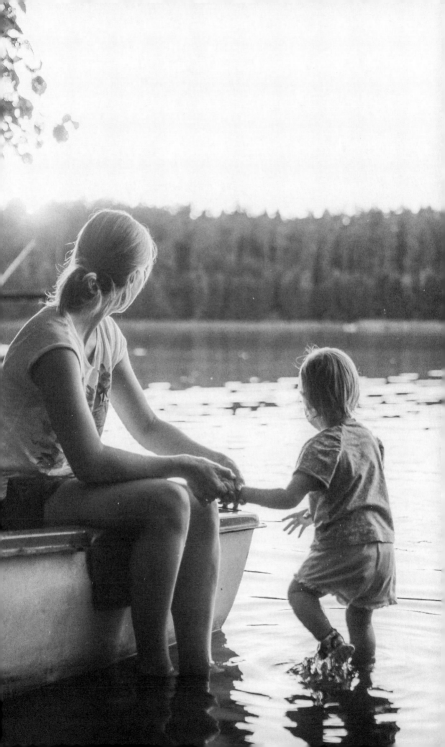

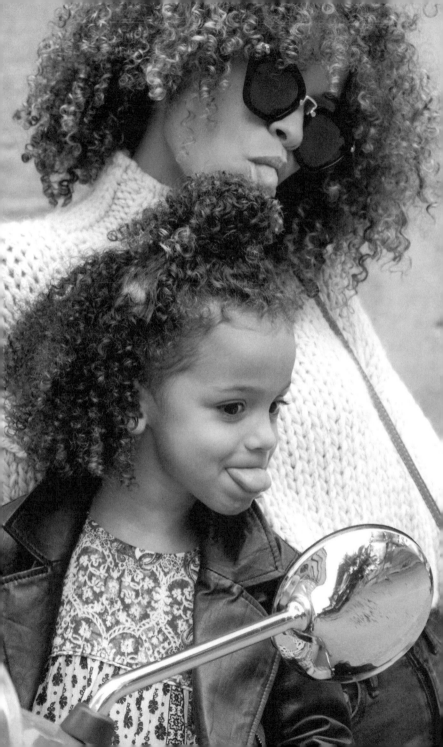

Self-Respect

At a parents' meeting, a primary school teacher I know asked, 'Imagine your child is twenty and wants to go travelling abroad. What qualities do you think they will need in order to cope when they're far away from home?'

The parents put themselves in their children's shoes and suggested 'self-belief' and 'self-respect'.

Then one father said, 'I keep telling my son he should have more self-confidence. But it does no good.'

When the teacher told me this story, I thought about how the father could foster confidence and self-respect in his son. The answer is not simply to tell children to gain confidence and have self-respect, but to lead by example. Self-respect is best learned from parents who embody this quality themselves.

Self-respect is the ability to accept and protect yourself, to forgive your mistakes and to have a little self-belief. Having self-respect allows us to maintain boundaries: when we have self-respect we expect others to treat us with dignity, and we step away from them when they don't.

Self-respect leads to resilience. It gives us the inner resources to manage the harsh words or behaviour of others, so we can respond appropriately, and remain strong emotionally.

Why is self-respect so important?

If we have a healthy sense of self, we can accept ourselves with all our flaws and failings. We know we are imperfect; when we fail we show resilience by having confidence that we could do better next time. We can also safeguard ourselves and define our own boundaries. If we know that we are not perfect, we can accept and respect other people and their imperfections too.

Giving children self-respect

Adults show children how to respect themselves through their own behaviour, so it is vital that as a parent you respect yourself and have confidence within your leadership role in the family. Children need their parents and carers to be leaders, not pals or partners. But getting the balance of authority and intimacy right within the context of a loving family can often be difficult for parents in practice.

Children's whims

When I talk to parents about respect in the family home, they often say things like, 'I have no problem getting respect at work, but it's much harder with the children.' If I ask them why they think this is, they often say that they don't like being firm with children, or that their relationship with their children feels dependent on giving the children their own way, and on being relaxed rather than setting boundaries.

Trying to please our children can lead to asking too often what they want: what do they want to eat, to wear, to buy, to do. Fulfilling children's wishes can become paramount within the family as a whole. I believe this kind of family pattern will undermine our efforts to earn our children's respect, and to model self-respect for them.

Don't let yourself be manipulated

If we try to ingratiate ourselves with our children, we can easily be manipulated. If we always ask children their preferences, they come to believe that they rule the roost, and this in turn will create frustrations for us.

Consider a mother who arrives at the supermarket to discover that her daughter's favourite brand of breakfast muesli is not in stock. The mother is immediately worried, picturing her daughter making a terrible scene the next morning. What makes this situation stressful for the mother is her belief that getting the 'right' muesli will guarantee her daughter's happiness. But happiness does not depend on a bowl of muesli. We need the confidence not to be guided by our children's whims. Family lives led by an attempt to avoid children's tantrums are often, indeed, unhappy. Children are learning how to balance their preferences with other people's needs and with the situation in hand. We can help with this by not fulfilling their wishes every time. If, as parents, we have a sense that we must meet children's demands constantly to ensure a peaceful family life, we are teaching them how to manipulate us, and thus how to manipulate others. When we have confidence in ourselves and our choices, we inspire confidence in our children.

Aggression in children

Parents sometimes complain to me that their children are aggressive: they hit, bite or scratch other children. When I ask the parents if their children are aggressive towards them too, the answer is often yes. The father of a two year old answered, 'Only sometimes,' before hurrying to add, 'but we don't really mind. Our main concern is that he shouldn't hit other children.'

Many parents say nothing when their children attack them, feeling they'd rather the children took out their aggression on them than on others.

But we are our children's role models, and if we have so little self-respect that we let ourselves be hit, our children will see us as victims. They will keep going, challenging us to establish limits and to model establishing limits for them. It is important to stand firm and state clearly what is not acceptable.

Parents show the way

Children are learning. As learners, they need parents who demonstrate expectations about behaviour clearly and immediately. Even if children do something naughty 'as a joke', make it clear when they have gone too far.

Imagine, for example, a three year old who runs around a restaurant pretending his breadstick is a sword. He is having great fun imagining himself a knight, but then he climbs up onto his father's knee and hits him in the face with his 'sword'. The breadstick breaks and scratches his father's cheek.

We might say 'He's only playing' and make light of it, but in this scenario, even if only in a small way, someone has been hurt during play. It is a natural impulse to excuse our children's behaviour, yet they need to know when they have hurt somebody. In a situation like this, I would suggest encouraging the boy to reflect on his behaviour, and demonstrating how to be more gentle. Ask him to play with his 'sword' away from the tables and other people.

You only gain respect if you respect and value yourself

Can children respect us if we do not respect, protect and define ourselves? Telling children, 'Stop that. I don't like it,' sends out a clear message to them when they have gone too far, and receiving that message can be a relief for them.

When I said this to a father I know, he replied, 'Well, I can tell you how my son will react to me saying stop: he'll just laugh at me.'

I'm sure that we have all had our children react to us with laughter when we are trying to be serious with them. It is in children's nature to test whether adults are authentic, whether we will stand up for what we say and follow through – not only in words but by expressing with our body language, tone of voice and actions that we really mean what they say. If our children refuse to take us seriously, we need to get serious with them and clearly, unambiguously communicate what we expect from them.

I like to think of the trembling aspen and the oak tree: use the oak tree as your inspiration when your children are trying to push your boundaries or manipulate you or hurt you. Stand fully upright with your feet planted firmly on the floor like a thousand-year-old oak rooted strongly in the earth. You will notice that you feel stronger simply by being physically upright.

In this position, look your child in the eyes. If they turn their head away – which children tend to do if directly confronted – say: 'Please look at me.' Repeat this until they do look at you, because your child will only realise that you really do mean what you say if you establish eye contact. And then say firmly what change in behaviour you expect.

Authority and clear communication

Try following these five steps when involved in a conflict with children:[6]

1. *Complete attentiveness:* Don't multi-task. Be fully present.
2. *Address children by name:* Use their own name and speak firmly.
3. *Eye contact:* Look children in the eyes.
4. *State clearly what you want:* Tell the child exactly what this is about, for instance: 'You must stop hitting!'

And if the child doesn't listen, use rule 5:

5. *Be persistent:* Insist on what you ask for and don't give up.

Clear, unambiguous body language works better than a thousand words. And during puberty it will be needed fairly often. Once you are used to it, it is far preferable to moaning at your children.

Of course, don't feel discouraged if it takes a few goes to get the hang of this. Remember, self-respect is acknowledging that we are not perfect and that life is an ongoing learning process. Parenthood, with all its challenges, offers us many opportunities to develop new approaches!

Are we belittling ourselves?

Parents often ask why their children aren't confident. Others are angry because their children speak to them dismissively. It can be illuminating to step back and consider whether we in fact talk about ourselves in dismissive terms, or whether we are habitually criticising ourselves and others, perhaps just at a low level:

'Oh, look how daft I am.' 'These people have no idea…' Owning up to mistakes is a strength, but constantly belittling ourselves is undermining, and creates an undermining picture for our children. And giving others the benefit of the doubt creates a culture of respect more broadly. If we need greater respect from our children, and we want them to respect themselves, the first task is cultivating genuine self-respect.

Being able to say no

When we say no to our children, we are teaching them how to say no and when it's appropriate. Here is an example I saw recently:

A five year old was with his mother at the playground, where his favourite thing is the Wendy house. On this day, there were two older boys in there. The little boy went into the Wendy house to play, but they scared him away. He ran off and the bigger boys chased him. His mother watched with concern but didn't want to step in too quickly. And then she saw her child turn around suddenly and firmly, stretch his hand out and call: 'Stop it! No!'

The two older boys stopped, and one said to the other, 'Come on, let's leave him alone.'

Later, when only the little boy could hear her, his mother said, 'Well done. You stood up for yourself today.'

This mother knew from the way her son said 'Stop it!' that he had learned his self-protective behaviour from her own.

Enjoy your own interests

Nowadays, modern life has so many pressures, as parents we often don't have the time to do the things we love, especially activities that don't fit in easily with family life. But children need to see us taking care of ourselves and pursuing our own aims. This is part of maintaining our own sense of self-worth, and thus of modelling self-respect. Children also need some space to find their own way, and parents who are very involved with them, even dependent on them, can be felt as a burden.

Even if I have very little time for major activities, I find it makes a big difference to my day if I set my alarm ten minutes earlier and have some 'me time' before everyone else gets up – just a little bit of stretching and a moment for reflection. I can find myself drawing on these moments later in the day: a bit of time to ourselves is sustaining.[7]

I also find it strengthening to look back on my day in the evening. I try to recall a positive experience, something that went well. Sometimes I write it down. Remembering good moments becomes a habit.

By being attentive to ourselves, by treating our own needs as important, we lay the ground for children to develop their own self-respect. We give them an authentic example to follow.

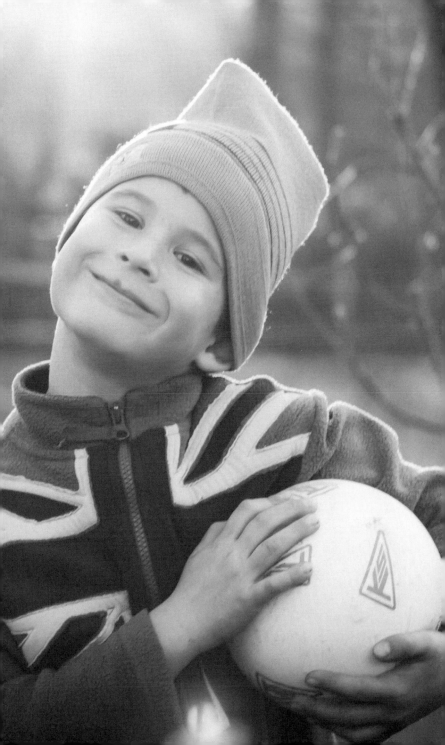

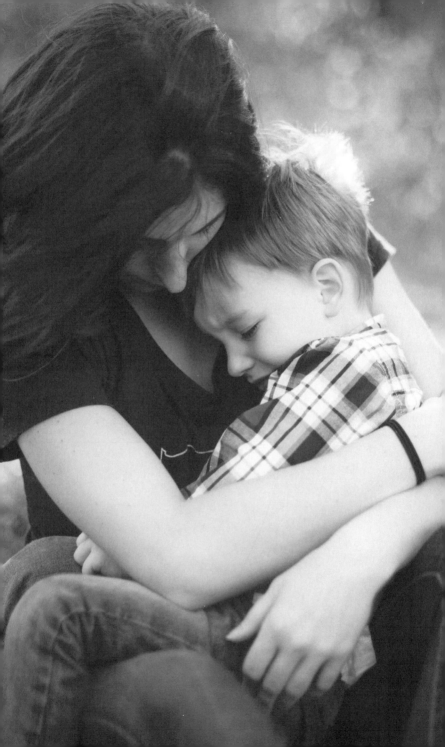

Empathy

A mother had a bad cold and lay on the sofa in the living room wrapped in blankets. There was no one around to look after her lively three-year-old and five-year-old boys, so she asked them if they could play especially quietly today. It worked! The children showed their gentlest sides: they immersed themselves in their play without any quarrelling or noise. Now and then, one came over and stroked his mother, gave her a kiss or brought her his favourite cuddly toy. The five year old said, 'I'll look after you.'

Some people might think the children in this example are unusual, or that this is an unrealistic depiction. But when I ask parents who have been in a similar situation, they say that when times are rough, if you talk to children clearly about what you feel and what you need, they can surprise you with their kindness and understanding.

Sensing how other people are feeling

All children have the ability to sense how other people are feeling and to recognise those feelings within themselves. And they can respond to others accordingly. Developmental psychologists tell us that this is because we have 'mirror neurones' in our brains.[8] Yet, while we are all equipped with mirror neurones, our natural capacity for sympathy or empathy can thrive or wither, depending on whether it is encouraged. We can all train and strengthen our ability to empathise with others.

How can empathy be nurtured, strengthened and practised?

As with self-respect, children best learn empathy when adults around them display this quality. Children perceive with great clarity what parents, carers and teachers model for them. Every day offers us plenty of opportunities to practise empathy – and it starts with taking our children's feelings seriously.

Allowing children to show their feelings

Would we prefer for our children to show what they feel, or would we prefer them to be tougher and more self-contained? How do we respond, for instance, if a young child is afraid of something – say, the doctor or dentist? Adults will often make light of children's concerns, saying dismissively, 'Oh, it'll be fine.' But does this allow for our children to have a different experience – an experience that is not fine? Or perhaps when our daughter's best friend moves away, we might try to comfort her by saying, 'There are lots of other nice children at school.' Or what if a beloved guinea pig dies – we might say, 'Never mind, we'll get you another one.'

Showing empathy

Children experience many troubling situations. In those situations, their powers of empathy will mature if adults engage with their feelings. Try addressing them and their feelings directly. If they are feeling afraid in the doctors' surgery, take them in your arms and be honest: 'Yes, the injection will hurt a little.' And then give physical support and comfort: 'But I'm here and I'll look after you.'

Or try to share their feelings if their best friend moves away: 'Yes, I know how sad you are now your best friend lives so far away. I can see you miss her.'

And if a guinea pig dies, don't replace it straight away with another one, while your children are still grieving. Show understanding: 'Yes, he was such a lovely guinea pig, wasn't he? Let's make a little grave for him and say goodbye.'

Acknowledging feelings as real helps children to name them, and to be OK with their feelings, even if they are not positive ones. And it helps them to perceive and acknowledge others' feelings too.

Managing conflict between children

How do we respond when one child hits or hurts another? As adults we often intervene by asking, 'Who started it? Why did you do this?' We make judgements and mete out punishments. It takes a little time and perspective to step back and consider whether we are being just. Often we witness only the attack and do not know whether it was provoked.

To deal with conflicts between children, I suggest the following approach to avoid the trap of injustice. First, say: 'Stop. We don't hit people.' Then attend to the child who was hit. We can empathise with the injury by saying, 'Goodness, that must have hurt!' And then we can say to the child who struck the blow, 'Come on, let's blow away the sore place you gave her.' Genuinely puff on the sore spot, so you are drawing attention to the soreness with actions as well as words.

Usually this will be enough to calm the children and bring a kind of reconciliation. Through this sympathetic example, children learn that whatever went on, whoever was right or wrong, if we empathise with hurt, things can be made better again.

Showing children how to apologise

The previous example is a good way to resolve conflicts between children, but situations in public places, where other people – including adults – might become involved, can be more difficult to manage. Let's consider the following scene:

A seven-year-old boy was at the park with his dad on a Sunday afternoon. Suddenly he picked up a stone and threw it at a family sitting on a bench nearby. 'Hey!' cried the father of the family. 'Stop that! You could hurt someone!'

The seven year old's dad simply told his son: 'Go over and say sorry.' The boy complied, offering a 'Sorry' with no eye contact or any other sign of remorse. Then he walked away.

In this scenario, the boy was going through the motions, but learned nothing about empathy. This often happens when we instruct our children to say 'sorry': they say the word but do not really understand the other person's feelings or what they have done wrong.

Children need adults who help them learn from their mistakes. When I imagine an alternative way for the boy's father to deal with this situation, I wonder whether the father could walk across to the family with his son, look them in the eye himself, and say, 'I'm very sorry about this.' His manner would show he was engaged and sympathetic rather than just paying lip service. In this way the father would show his son how to say sorry and mean it.

Then the father could take his son aside and, just between themselves, appeal to his feelings: 'What would it be like if someone suddenly threw a stone at you?' And if his son was defensive or reluctant to answer, he could persist, saying, 'Think for a moment, how would you feel?' Asking children to think about how their actions affect other people can help awaken their sense of empathy.

Laughter at someone else's expense

What if the hurtful thing your children are doing is laughing, rather than throwing a stone? Here is another scenario:

A mum and dad were out walking with their two children when they saw a man with crutches. They noticed he had only one leg. One of the children called out, 'Look at that funny man!' and then both began laughing loudly.

The parents said (quietly so that only the children could hear it), 'Stop that now. There's absolutely nothing to laugh at! Why do you think the man only has one leg? He might have had a bad accident. Do you think he should sit at home in a chair all the time? It's very brave of the man to come outside and walk with his crutches, and not funny at all.'

Later on, the older child told his parents, 'It wasn't really me laughing before; it was just something inside me. I didn't really want to laugh at all.'

By immediately putting a stop to their children's insensitive laughter, these parents have made it clear that this is an inappropriate reaction. They are teaching their children to consider the man's situation. The older child has clearly taken his parents' words to heart and reflected on why he reacted the way he did.

Empathy is a core value

Teaching children they must make the effort to understand what other people are feeling is an essential part of parenting and education. Empathy is a core value that makes human interaction and community possible. It is important for the mental health of every child to cultivate empathic behaviour, especially because they can often encounter a lack of it in daily life.

Children will see a lot of behaviour on screen, for example, that is far from empathetic. Even children whose screen use is limited will witness casual violence and abuse from time to time, because these elements of popular culture are so pervasive. As parents, we cannot alter the world, but we can take a stance. If you say, 'It's just a film, but I don't like what that character is doing,' your children will recognise that your views on empathy are consistent. Hearing your position can help them comprehend a confusing world.

The neuroscientist Manfred Spitzer says TV programmes that use physical pain for entertainment purposes will slowly erode our capacity for empathy. 'The reality is that this has an effect on viewers.'[9] Being aware of this can inspire us to reassert the value of empathy when confronted with violent images.

Avoiding negativity

We can set a strong example for children if we break the common habit of making constant negative comments on others. I'm thinking of all those little inattentive remarks about someone else being in the wrong, or judgements on how other people look or behave. To develop more empathy in ourselves and in our children, we can focus on the positive: always look out for what someone else did well and praise them for it.

Rudolf Steiner's 'positivity exercise', which is one of the six 'supplementary exercises', is helpful.[10] When we are confronted with an object or situation that is apparently completely negative or ugly, Steiner challenges us to find something positive in it. This doesn't mean denying the negative, or becoming uncritical, it is about recognising that buried in the negative there must be some positive – perceiving the multiple aspects of all experience.

Telling stories

Audiobooks are great, but there is something very special for children about being read to by their own family members. Children thrive in the comfort of your presence and in your engagement with them and the story. This engagement also helps to teach them empathy.

It can be frustrating when children want more and more stories at bedtime when you're trying to settle them. I suggest telling them in advance that there is only going to be *one* story today. But then tell it with real inner involvement. Put your heart into it, feel what you're reading. Keep making eye contact, and pause now and then to let your children say something or ask a question. Reading with involvement can create a wonderful feeling of connection, and it will help bedtime stories feel less of a chore and more a mutual pleasure.

If your children demand another story straight away, perhaps their own feelings weren't fully involved in the first. Try asking about it: 'What happened in that story? Do you remember what so-and-so did? And what happened next?' Or, the next day, encourage your children to paint of picture of the story. This will help them absorb what they've heard. It's not the quantity of reading that counts, but the quality of engagement.

Fairy tales

Once your children are old enough to understand slightly more complex narratives, try reading them fairy tales or folk tales, such as those collected by the Brothers Grimm.[11] But don't censor them! Many parents are reluctant to include the 'cruelties' that figure in some of these stories, or the 'bad passages', as I've heard them called. Don't sanitise them. All the difficulties, hopes and wishes of the central characters are a journey through the world of feelings. While children follow the ups and downs of the plot, they empathise with the good. The good eventually triumphs, rewarding their empathy. Folk tales assist emotional development.

Heroic deeds

Often children breathe a sigh of relief when the hero or heroine triumphs at the end of a story. This shows their capacity for empathy: the triumph of good touches and moves their souls. Children may want to speak more about a story they've heard, and they may include it in their play. Imagine what was happening inside for the little boy in this scene:

A four and a half year old walked through a wood talking repeatedly about what will happen 'when the witch comes'.

'I'll knock her down!' he said eagerly. He got a stick and thrust the imaginary witch away. 'And then she'll fall in the stream, won't she?' he asked his mother. 'And she won't be able to get out again.'

'No, she won't get out again, you're right,' his mother replied.

The little one was deeply content at the thought that he himself could conquer evil. Children want to feel this.

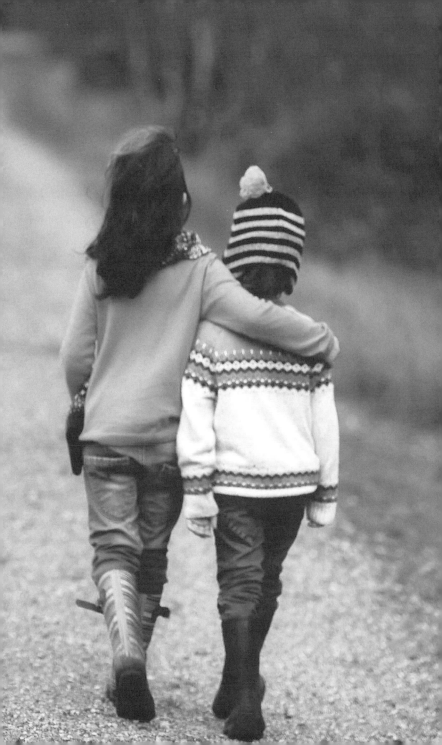

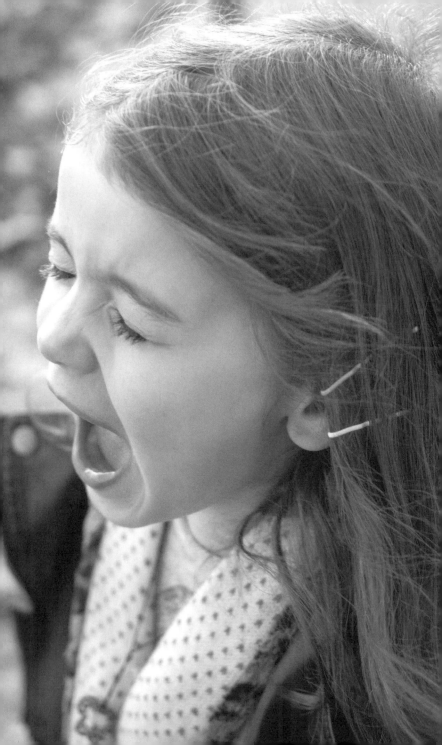

Capacity to Tolerate Frustration

Talking with a group of parents, I asked them, 'Who is the boss at home?'

One replied immediately, 'Well, it certainly isn't me!'

Everybody laughed.

I tend to find that this is true for most parents I talk to. We all want our children to like us and to think of us as their friends. Yet there is a danger that this approach sends out the message 'No conflicts, please.' Can we consider the idea that this is exactly what invites conflict between parents and children?

A united front

Sometimes two parents disagree on how best to deal with children, and conflicts arise between them. Consider this scene:

A mum and dad are sitting with their daughter on a train. The child starts drumming her shoes on the opposite seat.

Her dad says, 'Please take your shoes off the seat.' When she keeps on doing it, he repeats what he's just said – and she immediately starts crying.

Her mum comforts her, stroking her back, saying, 'There, there, he didn't mean to be nasty.'

The child sobs for a little longer – and then she goes back to kicking the opposite seat.

And the dad says nothing.

The mum has prioritised their daughter's present mood over the dad's attempts to make her behave. If this pattern takes over, there is a risk the dad's role in his daughter's upbringing could be minimised. This is a commonplace family dynamic and, of course, the roles can easily be reversed.

If, as parents, we can see eye to eye in important areas of upbringing, it will help immensely with raising our children. When one parent says one thing and the other something else, children soon learn that they will get their own way by making a fuss. These disagreements between parents, while common, can disturb family equanimity and do more harm than good for children.

Giving in to a dissatisfied child

If parents are always trying to please children, and if children learn that they can bend their parents to their will, they will come to believe their own desires are the most important – and they can have major tantrums when they don't get their way.

Many parents tell me that their children want to call the shots. When I asked one mother how she responded to this attitude from her son, she said, 'His father and I usually give in – we don't like having arguments. To begin with, we thought he'd grow out of it. But now he's at school the teacher complains he is always at the centre of conflicts, and we'd like that to stop.'

Being in charge

Our children are not machines, so we can't switch off bad behaviour. The only real remedy is to take control as parents and educate our children. We need to make it clear that we are in charge – as we are when we drive a car, for example.

We would never let our children drive a car. Adults always sit in the driving seat. No tantrum or any other fuss would convince us to let our children drive. So when we're in the car we have clear, unbending rules. In our daily childcare, we can take charge in the same way.

To reduce conflict in the long run, rather than in the immediate moment, I suggest parents clearly assign roles: we are the bosses, not our children.

One mother at a workshop with me shifted uncomfortably on her chair: 'The boss?' she said. 'That sounds so stupid. I don't want to be the boss.' But the word itself doesn't matter. What matters is that we as parents realise that we are the only ones who can really take responsibility and make the decisions. 'Decision-maker,' the mother said when I suggested this alternative. 'Yes, that sounds better. I'd rather be the decision-maker.'

However we think of ourselves as parents, it is important that we give our children clear guidance, and not the other way round. In the example of the girl kicking her shoes against the seat, all that was needed was a clear instruction: 'Please take your shoes off the seat!' The girl's father was not being nasty; he was teaching her an important social rule.

And if children shout and don't do what we ask, then remember the five steps for clear communication and authority from the chapter on self-respect. Stay credible instead of giving in.

Clear rules

We can avoid many daily conflicts if there are clear agreements and rules for situations that have previously proved difficult: for example, mealtimes or bedtimes. Sit down with your partner and have a calm conversation about rules you could have in your household. Questions to ask could include:

What rules should we have?
Which situations need rules?
How should we apply them?
When should we apply them?

The next step is to tell children what the rules are, reiterate them so they can be put into practice and – most importantly – tirelessly keep to them. Both parents need to stick to what they have decided together for the rules to be a success.

Testing our consistency

Children wouldn't be children if they didn't keep on testing whether rules really apply. I have heard parents describe a scenario like the one below time and again:

Dinner is over and the table has been cleared. A girl asks her dad, 'Can I go and play?'

Her dad has an idea what's going on. He asks her, 'And what did Mummy say?'

The girl turns her head away and Dad smiles. It turns out that Mum had just called her to come and brush her teeth.

With the neutral question, 'And what did Mummy/Daddy say?' we can prevent children playing us off against each other and causing conflicts.

Saying no when necessary

It is fine to say no when the situation demands it, but of course it can be difficult to refuse children something that they want, so I suggest practising. Next time your children make a fuss because they want something they can't have, show your ability to deal with conflict by saying warmly yet firmly, 'No.' And if they protest, 'But we want it!' a good answer is, 'You might want it, but I have said no, and no means no.'

It is perfectly normal for children to oppose us. They want to challenge their parents and test whether we are credible.

Be steadfast

When children become frustrated, it can be difficult to cope with their distress. But remember to stay clear and focused and tell them, 'I mean what I say.'

In the long term, this enables children to deal with disappointment, to respect others and to self-regulate. No one else, not even their parents, can relieve them of these tasks. Let them feel frustration. The objection that this is heartless, that 'I can't let my child cry,' is exactly the trap into which we often fall. We want the crying to stop and so we give in. Conflict and friction are avoided in the short-term. But remember that friction can be positive: to extend the metaphor, where there is friction, there is also warmth and contact.

Friction is necessary

When we experience friction with our children, we are in real contact with them, and thus we give them safety and security. Children are then able to develop emotionally, instead of staying at the infantile stage into school years and beyond.

I believe that people cope better with life if they have learned from an early age that things cannot always go their way. Parents must constantly balance children's individual needs with the needs of the family as a whole. Children do not have the oversight to do this themselves. On those occasions when we see that the needs of the whole will be better served by refusing a child's wishes, we do best to say no to the child: we are ensuring the smooth, balanced running of family life, and also giving the child a real and valuable experience.

I once heard a father speaking to his son: 'I'm saying no because I love you and so I'm willing to challenge you. If you didn't matter to me, I wouldn't bother. I'd make life easier for myself.' Being prepared to enter into conflict shows children they are worth struggling with.

No one can win all the time

When we play games with our children, it's tempting to let them win, because we believe it will make them happy. But it's also important for children to learn that they are not perfect.

A father once told me, 'I always used to let our son win until a friend pointed out that this gives children a completely false idea of the world: they come to believe that success will come to them automatically. It had got a bit like that in our case. So next time we had a running competition, I ran faster than my son on purpose. He got in a complete rage. And I told him, "No one can win all the time."'

Everyone makes mistakes

No one is infallible. We all make mistakes: they are normal, human and instructive. Mistakes give us opportunities to develop. If we are capable of handling frustration and conflict, we can acknowledge mistakes – and the moment we do, the mood lightens. Observe it for yourself.

Our children, and our partners too, will feel we have made a big gesture if we acknowledge a mistake. Next time you have done the wrong thing, look them in the eye and say, 'I overreacted. What I said was pretty stupid and unfair. I'm sorry.' This has a healing effect and creates real intimacy.

Frustration first aid

The following 'first aid' can be helpful if your own frustration feels like it is boiling over. Say, 'I'll be back in a moment!' and leave the room. This will stop you overreacting and doing or saying something you will regret. It also stops you issuing threats you cannot follow through. Drink a glass of water. Feel the soles of your feet. Breathe deeply for a minute or two. Then, refreshed, return to the room and tell your child once again, clearly and firmly: 'I'm waiting for you to do this. Now do it, please.' Stay close by your child to give them security, and remember the value of humour.

Conciliatory farewell

It is well worth trying to have a loving farewell each morning, especially if there has been an argument. No one can concentrate properly when they have separated from a family member in stress and anger. I often hear parents say things like, 'I need an hour or so to calm down again after I get to work.'

The same distress happens for our children. Even if they are young, they feel the effects of arguments deeply, and may worry that their parents don't like them. Try to end disputes as people leave the house for the day. At this point children need the blessings and warm farewell of their parents. That way they can feel the arguments were only about what they *did*, not *who they are*. Reassure them that they are loved.

Likewise, it is important to make peace at bedtime. However angry a conflict has been, children thrive best if they can take a sense of reconciliation into sleep. Try telling them, 'Today is over, and tomorrow, things can go better. Sleep well. Mummy and Daddy love you.' We can never tell our children too often that we love them.

When parents take charge, and when we show ourselves to be authentic, humane and capable of learning, we release ourselves and our children from the conflict zone of intransigence, stubbornness and perfectionism. The behaviour we model as parents in conflict situations is far more important than all our words and warnings.

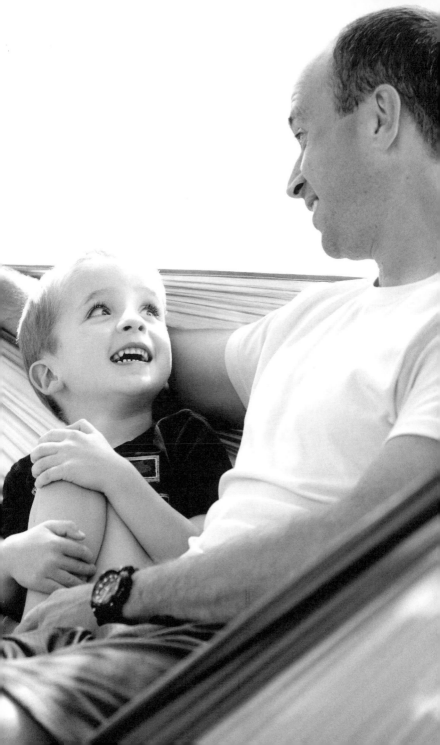

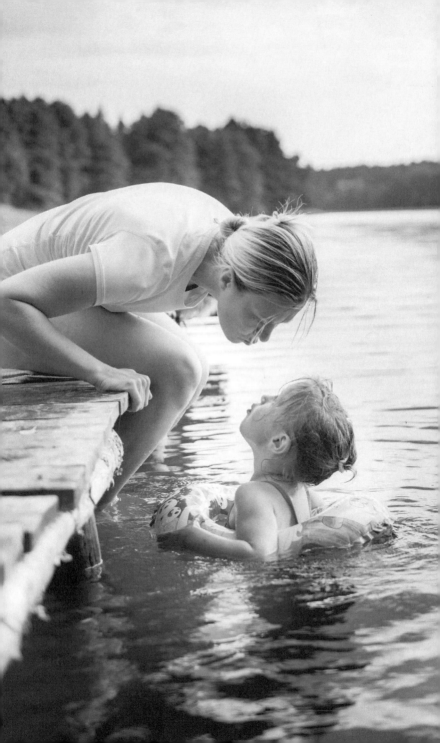

Independence

'Our son dawdles so much in the morning. It feels like we're always nagging him to get ready faster and packing his bag for him so he isn't late for school,' said the parents of a ten-year-old boy.

I'm sure this is a familiar scenario for many parents, but take a minute to think about it. Is it our job as parents to relieve our children of all responsibilities? Do they always have to be helped? It might seem that children need our assistance so that they don't get into trouble, but perhaps our insistence on stepping in creates the problem in the first place.

Children want to do things for themselves

When children are struggling it's natural to want to help, but actually they need to learn to do things themselves. In fact, even very young children *want* to do things themselves; our 'help' sometimes hinders them – and, in the process, robs them of the delight of discovering that they are capable. Consider this example:

A six-month-old baby was lying on a blanket on the ground, trying to grasp a toy just out of reach. She stretched and concentrated. She had almost got there. But then her mum bent down and handed it to her.
When I asked the mother why she did this, she said, 'I just wanted to help.'

Does this sound familiar? The mum's efforts are well meaning, of course, yet in the long term they are not helpful. We have to let our children stretch in all ways, not relieve them of every effort.

Naturally we can do things quicker and better than an infant. We can reach objects more easily and build higher towers. And, of course, if we do them ourselves, the housework and cooking get done more speedily – and the same goes for dressing children. We have good intentions when we do these things, but in the process, we disadvantage our children because we prevent them from challenging themselves.

Over-caring blocks children's independence

Nowadays many four or five year olds, and even older children, are not yet able to dress themselves or put on their shoes. Children older than we might expect are still pushed in buggies. We parents do all the housework and make packed lunches for our twelve year olds.

If asked why they do this, parents usually say, 'It speeds everything up.' But there's a high price to pay. If we relieve our children of all responsibilities because it's easier or more practical for us, we are teaching them that we don't expect them to make an effort. There is a risk that they may fail to develop in age-appropriate ways, making them dependent on us for longer than they need to be.

Children love to help

Given the chance, children love to lend a hand, and they will benefit from the fact that we trust them to join in and be useful. Think about this example:

A grandmother was looking after her four-year-old grandson for the afternoon. 'Would you like to make an apple cake?' she asked him.

His eyes lit up. 'Yes please, Granny!'

He helped his grandmother weigh out all the ingredients and sieve the flour into the bowl. He watched his grandmother crack an egg into the bowl, and she let him do the next one himself. He mixed all the ingredients together.

She peeled and cored the apples while the little boy stood on a stool beside her. He had a chopping board and a knife and was allowed to chop the quartered apples and put them in the saucepan. He was completely absorbed in this.

'You're doing that very well,' his grandmother said. 'You must be a great helper for Mummy and Daddy!'

'No,' he said. ' They don't let me do anything!'

Trust and encouragement

Children develop their abilities by doing. From a young age children have a natural joy in doing, and we can build on this. They need encouragement and trust. Tell them, 'You can do that yourself. You're old enough now.'

Think about what you let your children do. What skills do you encourage them to develop? Are they given tasks around the house? Or, like so many others, would you say that they only help occasionally, when they feel like it? Don't underestimate your children, and support them in activity rather than passivity.

Involvement reduces boredom

Children being 'difficult' may be the result of not having enough responsibility, or not feeling part of the household. Consider this example:

A couple consulted me for advice about their four year old because he fidgeted throughout the evening meal and chucked leftovers on the floor as soon as he was tired of eating.

When I asked if he helped to prepare the meal, his parents said no. I asked them if he buttered his own bread and the parents said, 'No, he doesn't.'

'Why not?'

'He's so young we always do it for him. I suppose he could butter his own bread actually. We'll give it a try,' they replied.

A few days later they were very pleased to report that their son was so busy buttering his own bread at meals that he no longer fidgeted or threw things.

Was this child really being 'difficult' or was he simply bored? When children help to prepare food, it takes on a different meaning for them. Once this boy became more engaged with what he was eating, his behaviour immediately improved. What other tasks could we give our children to engage them, make them feel valued, and capture their attention?

'Let me!'

Even very young children vehemently announce that they want to do things themselves. Why not take them at their word? It only takes a few more minutes if we encourage our children to dress themselves. Try saying, 'You can start it off, I'll do the rest.' It's worth giving them the chance to prove themselves, because if they are prevented from following their impulses they will soon lose the will to try.

Give children the joy of helping when you're sweeping up, drying dishes, or loading and unloading the washing machine. Give them encouraging smiles and nods. This enhances their sense of importance, and children of all ages need to feel valued.

Household tasks

Children need regular household tasks, for example, helping in the kitchen, laying the table and clearing away after meals – and not just their own plate but everyone else's too.

There are other tasks around the home that children can easily help with: changing the duvet, sorting socks, watering flowers, cleaning shoes and much more. Discuss with children which ones they will do and then, to help them remember, write a list on a piece of paper and put it on a pin-board or the fridge. This saves unnecessary discussions. If children complain: 'I don't want to,' calmly and clearly point to the list and say, 'That's what we agreed, and that's what we'll do.'

Provide guidance

Of course children can't do everything themselves straightaway, but with a strong example to follow, they will even learn to deal with an accident themselves:

A boy tipped over his glass of milk. Rather than dash angrily for a cloth and clean up the milk himself, his father said, 'Come on, we'll mop it up together.'

With the boy's help, the father fetched a bucket and cloth, and together they mopped up, then washed and squeezed out the cloth.

The father said, 'Look, it's all fine again!' and the boy laughed.

By working together, the boy learned something, and he redeemed his own mistake, so he could feel OK about it.

Helping with school work

'It took me a long time,' said a mother in one of my workshops, 'to realise that I had made my daughter too dependent on me. Now I've stopped spending hours going over her school work with her while she sits there yawning. I told her that I've already passed my exams, and now it's up to her to pass hers.'

How can we respond if our children complain about their homework, saying, 'I can't do it. Can you do it for me?' Instead of giving in, try telling them that you'll support them but they must do it themselves.

Children's independence can be achieved much more easily by agreeing a clear structure for approaching their homework. Discuss this with them and let them write down the distinct stages legibly on a piece of paper, so that they really sink in:

1. Before sitting down to homework, get some exercise in the fresh air if possible.
2. Decide a fixed time for starting homework.
3. Always do homework in the same place.
4. Clear the table or desk before starting homework – put away toys, comics or devices so there are no distractions.
5. Make sure all necessary equipment (pencils, pens, worksheets) are set out before you start.
6. Parents could look at the homework book, and suggest that children start with the simpler tasks first and then move on to the harder ones. Encourage them and show interest but then let them get on with it themselves.
7. Be available but don't sit beside them or watch constantly. Have your own activities to get on with nearby. Tell them they can ask you if they have specific questions.

Encourage perseverance

Perseverance strengthens the will and develops skills. Encourage children to stick with their tasks, whether those are homework or hobbies. Children often start off pursuing new interests with great enthusiasm but then suddenly tire of them. Don't let them give up too easily. At the very point when things get harder they need someone who will spur them on and support them, helping them to keep going even though it's tough. See your role as encouragement rather than rescue. And, eventually, if their efforts pay off, you will see in their eyes how pleased they are at their achievements.

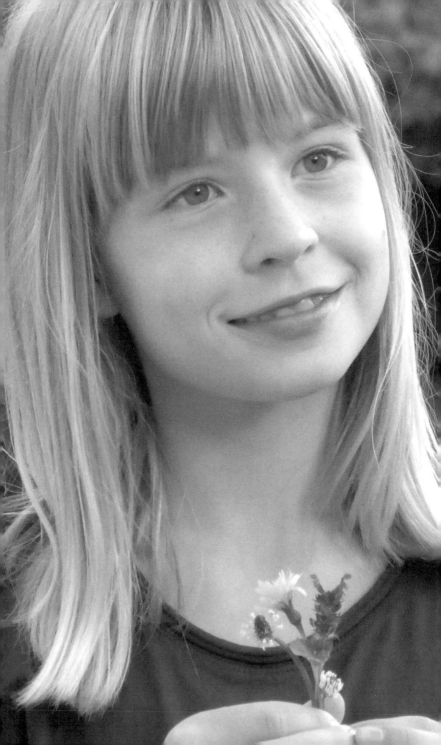

Gratitude

Showing gratitude and appreciation is essential to human life, and children need to learn the forms this takes in the social world around them. Knowing how to make requests politely and then acknowledge what others do for them smoothes our children's interactions with others. Every act of attentiveness is a bridge we build to reach other people. Greeting people, being friendly, giving a smile, taking leave of people – these small acts lead to strong relationships. Understanding the good that others bring us is essential to connection and inner wellbeing.

Setting an example

Children will follow our example if we always say 'thank you' when we receive something or when someone does something for us. Remember to also say thank you to children if they pass you something or fulfil a request.

Toddlers love to play please and thank you games:

'Will you please give me the ball?' called a father to his child, who had just learned to walk.

The little boy understood and brought him the ball, and gave his daddy a radiant smile too because he was so pleased to be asked politely.

'Thank you,' the father said. Then he gave the ball back to his son.

Then, 'Please can I have the ball again?' he asked.
And so it goes, back and forth.

This is a natural and relaxed way for little children to learn how to say thank you.

Saying please and thank you

If children never say please, then teach them. If, at mealtimes, for instance, your son calls out 'I want the butter!' show him how to ask in a friendlier way: 'May I have some butter, please?' Whenever children demand something rudely, repeat their request with a please.

Try to set a good example even in difficult situations. 'Even when I'm annoyed,' said one father I know, 'I always include a please. "Please don't speak to me like that." Or, "Please stop doing that."'

There is always time for a please. And, likewise, for a thank you.

A delicatessen assistant gave a two year old a sample of cheese. He took it without a word, so his mother said thank you for him.

At this, the little one called out 'Thank you!' too. He imitated her.

Words of welcome

'My child never greets me when I get home,' one father complained. 'He just stays in his room. Sometimes I wonder if anyone is pleased to see me!'

Other parents say their children don't like greetings, and make excuses for their behaviour: 'He's just a strong character.'

Sometimes parents make such statements proudly, but mutually appreciative behaviour needs conscious nurture in a family. When people know each other very well, there is a risk of taking one another for granted.

Greeting each other in an attentive and loving way is an excellent foundation for an appreciative family life. It shows we are genuinely glad of one another's presence. This starts with the first meeting in the morning – try to say 'Good morning' and 'How are you today?' rather than just a weary 'Hi' as you slip past each other. When someone comes home, greet them by name, with warmth and eye contact.

If children don't tend to greet people, then show them how to do so. Take them by the hand and say, 'Come on, let's say hello to Granny,' or whoever else it might be. Warm greetings tell other people they are important to us. They show we are grateful for and glad of others.

Good habits

At around four years old, children are able to say please and thank you, and they can greet people by themselves if they have seen this practised around them. And if they forget sometimes, we can gently remind them to do it next time.

Good habits are formed through experience and following good examples. Eventually, saying please and thank you and giving greetings become as habitual as teeth brushing. But the good example is essential. Constant chiding for forgetting manners, or constant prompting, quickly becomes empty. Demonstrate with actions rather than just insisting with words. And, most importantly, be polite and warm to your children. When children feel appreciated they are much more likely to appreciate others and to show this in their own words.

Gratitude for food

Nowadays, in the western world, we can buy food on every street corner. But we should remember that being able to sit down to a plate of food is a privilege; we should appreciate what we have.

Why not wait till everyone is ready before starting to eat, and then mark this with a little ritual honouring of our food? We can all hold hands to create a sense of community; we can look at one another and wish each other *bon appetit*. That's authentic, and children accept authentic things. Think about this example and whether this practice or something similar could be taken up in your household:

Two parents told me of their four year old. His kindergarten had a special ritual each day before lunch, and one evening at home when his parents were about to start eating, the boy said, 'Wait a moment!'

He put his fingers together and recited a little verse (by Christian Morgenstern):

Earth who gave to us this food,
Sun who made it ripe and good,
Dear earth, dear sun, by you we live,
Our loving thanks to you we give.

Since then, the boy's parents have adopted the verse as a family ritual. They say it with him at every meal.

Swearing

Parents at a workshop were complaining that their children swear.
'Do you ever swear yourselves?' I asked.
'We try not to,' said one mother.

Her husband chided, 'But just now when you were driving...'
'OK, yes, but the children weren't there.'

Swearing induces a negative mood. It expresses the opposite of gratitude and appreciation for others and for the world around us. If we expect children not to use swearwords, it is best never to swear ourselves. And that doesn't simply mean refraining in front of the children. It requires a shift in attitude.

Gratitude and respect for living things

How can we respond if children drag a cat by its tail or pull the legs off a fly? Children who do such things often look quickly at adults to gauge their reaction, so respond immediately. Stop them, and say, 'Treat other creatures as you would like to be treated.'

Follow through

A kindergarten group went out for a walk beside a flowering meadow. One of the girls started pulling the heads off flowers along the way.

One of the teachers, who had been at the kindergarten a long time, said to her newer colleague, 'Honestly, children have no respect for anything these days!'

Instead of replying, the newer teacher called out firmly, 'Hey, stop that! Flowers are living creatures too, let them flourish.'

The girl just laughed, and a few other children joined in.

But then the new teacher did something unexpected. She bent down and picked up the flower heads, saying, 'They're lovely. Let's not waste them. We can take them with us and look after them.' Without prompting, some of the children followed her example.

Back at kindergarten, the new teacher put the flower heads in a bowl of water. Placed on the dining table, they shone brightly for several days.

'That looks really beautiful,' said the very girl who had started pulling them off. Inside, something had changed for her.

Gratitude for all Creation is something we adults can cultivate in ourselves, and we can show children the values we live by. This can bring much healing and joy into the world.

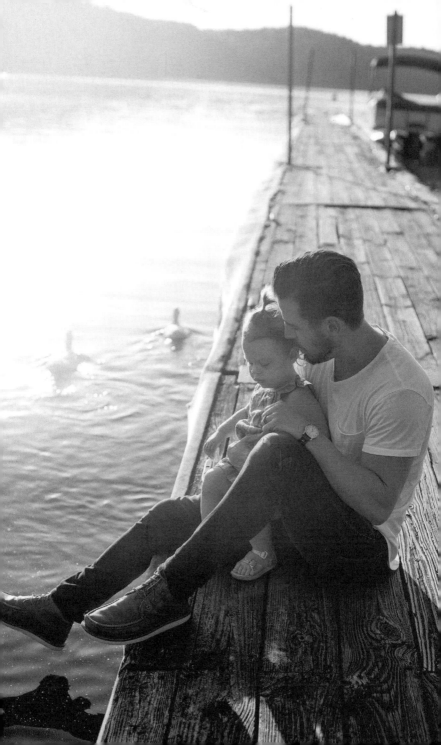

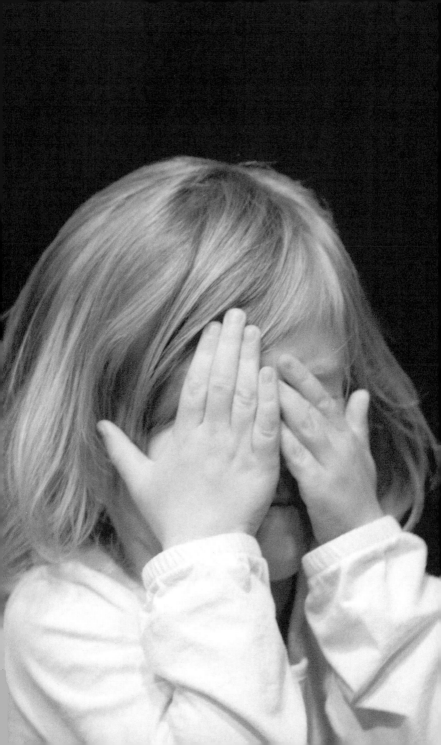

Truthfulness

When I ask parents what they feel is the worst thing their children could do, most tell me: lying.

One father I asked said, 'I get really furious when my daughter lies.'
'When was the last time she did?' I asked.
'She drew on the walls, but she pretended she hadn't – she said it was her younger sister.'
'And what did you do then?'
'I broke her pencils and sent her to her room.'
'And how did you feel afterwards?'
'Bad, of course. But I won't let her lie to me.'

No one likes being lied to

But are we ourselves always truthful or honest? Do we sometimes make promises we don't keep? If we tell children, 'We'll go to the playground later,' do we always go?

Adults get away with a lot. For instance, we might tell our children that the pasta sauce doesn't have any vegetables in it, even though we have hidden some finely chopped vegetables in it. Or, at the entrance to the zoo, we say, 'We'll tell them you're still five, so it won't cost anything to get in.'

Children often witness such untruths, and with them they receive the message that lying is acceptable. Naturally they will imitate the adults around them.

Children want to be honest

Unlike adults, children tend to be honest automatically, as long as they feel there is no reason to be afraid. Here is an example of parenting with an eye to future behaviour, as well as present behaviour:

A mother who is busy leaves her young daughter playing by herself in the living room. The mother hears something crash to the floor; shortly afterwards the little girl appears in the doorway looking glum.

'Mummy, look...'

The mother comes to the living room and sees her favourite vase in pieces. She is upset and cries, 'My beautiful vase! Oh no!'

Yet after she calms down, the mother says, 'Come on, we'll clear it up together.' And they do. Then she looks at her daughter and says, 'I am sad about the vase, but thank you for telling me straight away.'

The mother's positive message, 'Thank you for telling me straight away,' will make it easier for her daughter to tell the truth next time. On the other hand, parental 'inquisitions' create fear, which lead to distress. And everyone – big or small – reacts to such feelings by no longer daring to tell the truth.

Making things right again

Sometimes we adults can't help expressing displeasure at our children's behaviour, but it's important, after that initial reaction, that we avoid punishing them. Children don't learn anything from punishment. It is much more constructive to teach them to make things right again themselves. They need help and guidance in how to go about this, as in the example of the mother and the broken vase.

Similarly, the father whose daughter had drawn on the wall

could have painted over the drawings with her help. He could have found some large paper and asked his daughter to promise to use that in future.

Trust

Many parents complain that when they ask their children if they have brushed their teeth or washed their hands, they will say they have when they haven't. 'How do you know they haven't?' I asked one father.

'We check. We look in her mouth or check her hands to see if they smell of soap.'

'Why?'

'Well, I don't trust my child,' he said. 'She never does what she should.'

This might seem like a necessary intervention while children are young, but how long will it go on for? Imagine doing this day after day, month after month, year after year… Will we still be checking our children have washed their hands when they are twelve?

Something that is small to begin with, like checking up on the brushing of teeth, can become a bad habit for parents. For instance, a fifteen-year-old girl I know was distraught to find that her parents had been reading her personal diary. They said they read it in the interests of their daughter's safety; they wanted to check what she was doing. But spying on children is a violation of their dignity, and such parental mistrust will wreck family relationships. At some point we need to give up trying to control our children.

Practice, not control

'But,' parents ask me, 'how can we be sure our children are doing the right thing if we give up control?'

The answer is by practising instead. Adults usually under-estimate how important it is to continually practise daily activities with children, such as washing hands and brushing teeth. We can show them how we brush our teeth, how we wash and dry our hands and so on. Simply do it with them day after day, week after week, month after month, until they're ready for you to say, 'OK, you can do this by yourself now, can't you?'

If the child nods, look them in the eye and say, 'Good. Then from now on you'll do it on your own.' Remember to make eye contact: this makes an agreement solid.

If children are telling the truth, they will naturally look you in the eye. If they don't, try to delve a bit deeper.

When a boy gets back from playing at his friend's house, his trouser pocket is bulging. His mother says, 'What have you got there?'

'Oh, nothing.'

'But I can see something in your pocket.'

He reluctantly brings out a toy car.

'Where did you get that?'

'It's a present.'

The mother is dubious and pursues it further. 'Is it really a present?' she asks. 'Please look at me.'

The boy raises his head but doesn't look her in the eye.

His mother says again, 'Please look at me.'

Eventually the boy says, 'I didn't mean to take it...'

It becomes clear that the car wasn't given to the boy and has to be returned. The mother asks her son if he would like her to come with him, but he says he'd rather do it alone.

'And did he return it?' I asked.

The mother told me, 'I asked him if he had and he looked me in the eye, nodded vigorously, and said, "Yes".'

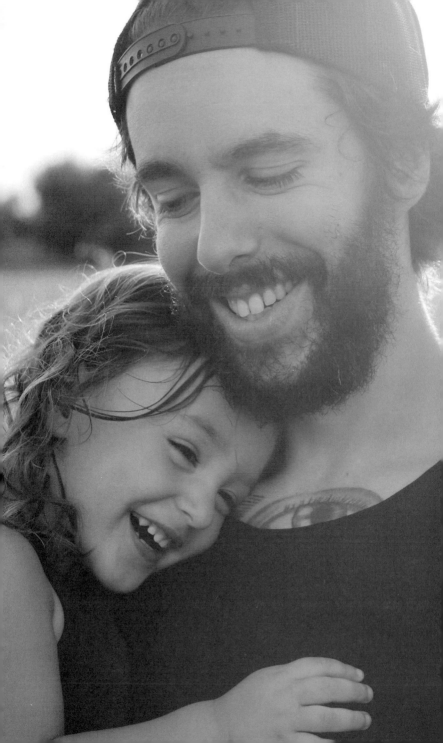

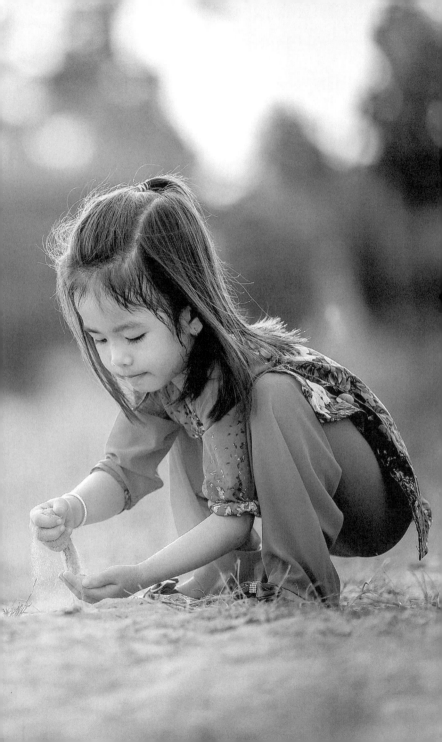

Interest in the World

Three things we still possess from Paradise: the stars of the night, the flowers of the day and the eyes of children.

The eyes of children are indeed precious, as the great poet Dante noted. Part of their preciousness is that looking into them will tell us immediately whether children are engaged, open and interested in the world, whether they can be fired with enthusiasm, or whether the opposite is true.

The shining eyes of children

I suggest that we take note of when children's eyes really shine. Is it when they are relieved of all effort? When everything happens as they demand? When they have shouted and got the sweets they want? When they are allowed to sit in front of a screen? When they are being 'entertained'?

If we observe carefully, we will find that children are not really made happy by such treats. Their eyes shine when they are actively engaged in something, when they are investigating or trying something out – in other words, when they are following their interest in the world outside themselves.

Having interest in the world is natural

People who are interested want to learn, discover and know something new – not because they are forced to, but out of their own curiosity. Children arrive in the world with this capacity. They are full of the joy of discovery and engaged by everything.

That is why it is so important to go out with children often and, rather than offering them everything on a plate, allow them to find things out for themselves. If they are allowed to, little children find astonishing things everywhere in the world: a leaf, a pebble, a pinecone. Everything they can pick up and hold is lifted for inspection and shown to us.

Interest needs to be shared

It is important to respond when children show us things. If we don't share in their interest, children's natural joy in discovery can be lost.

As giants, children come to earth,
Yet with every passing day,
A little of their power is lost,
As we shrink them in some way.[12]

If our behaviour is careless or dismissive, we can diminish our children's capacity for wonder.

'But that's the last thing we want,' parents say to me when I share this poem with them. 'We want them to enjoy the world and fulfil their potential!'

We can show our own outside interests to our children by speaking with them. Start chatting to infants as you go around together. Make sure you keep distractions to a minimum and avoid asking toddlers constantly, 'Do you want a banana? Would you like something to drink?' Instead, focus on the world around you.

And this is another reminder to avoid looking at your phone all the time. Concentrate on watching children in order to perceive them and their interests more intimately. That way the outing is more satisfying for everyone.

'Mummy, Mummy, look!' cried a two and a half year old while out for a walk. He had found a giant reed and was holding it up like a flag.

His mother replied, 'Hang on, wait a minute. Yes, stay like that!' She rummaged in her bag for her smartphone – she wanted to take a picture.

When she found the phone, she said, 'Now, do what you were doing just then. Yes, and laugh again like that!' The little one did it, but the moment had passed, and with it his enthusiasm.

How is the child feeling now? Or to put it another way, if we put ourselves in the shoes of this little world-explorer, what would we have wanted? When I asked this question at a parenting workshop, participants' deepest wishes bubbled up.

What children really want

'Look at me!'
'Be interested in me!'
'Listen to me!'
'Wonder with me!'
'Speak with me!'
Children want real attention; they want adults to see the miracles they discover. And that's why it is so important to respond for a moment at least: to give children a sense that what they have found is lovely and interesting. This affirmation encourages them to continue their ongoing interest in the world.

Our children seek contact with their most beloved possessions on earth: us, their parents. And they have many, many questions for us.

The capacity to question

'What is this called?'

'What's that?'

'Why is the person over there doing that?'

Some parents find their children's questions wearing and endless. A mother in a parenting workshop said, 'It winds me up when they keep on asking and asking.' Exercising patience can be tricky, but it is possible for us to step back and enjoy children's questions.

Think of it this way: the capacity to question is one of our most special human attributes. Someone who asks is interested in things and is in touch with their own inner development. It's worth observing the astonishing questions children ask. They are full of desire to know more about the world and everything in it.

'Why is the apple juice in the bottle yellow, but apples are white inside?' asked a six year old.

'That's a good question,' his parents reply. 'I wonder why we never thought of that before. Let's look it up in a book and try to find the answer.'

'Why? why? why?'

Children can ask 'why' till the cows come home. We won't always know the answer, but we can say, 'Let's find out.' Or hand the question back to them – and it is astonishing what profound answers children come up with.

'What happens to the sun when it goes down?' asks a four year old.

'What do you think?' asks his mother.

The little one replies, deeply satisfied, 'It goes to sleep!'

Keep conversing with children. By doing so, we are sustaining this fascinating capacity that children possess: to ponder something that interests them.

Try not to pacify children with devices

A couple go into a restaurant with their two-year-old son and give him a tablet to entertain him. 'At least we can eat in peace and talk to each other,' they say. The child sits spellbound by the artificial images. He does not say or ask anything: he stares at the screen in silence.

When something seems too good to be true, it usually is. In this example, what seems like an easy option for parents might actually harm their child's mental development. If we present children with ready-made entertainment, we deprive them of the chance to find things out for themselves. They can become accustomed to this continual distraction that is provided from the outside and lose their interest in the real, tangible world.

Further, Manfred Spitzer writes, 'We know that the foundations of addictive behaviour are laid in childhood and youth.'[13] Much of young children's interactions with screen-based entertainment can have similarities with addictive behaviour. What can we do to help address this problem?

There is much public debate today about supporting child development, but I particularly want to emphasise the importance of children's real interactions with their parents.

What is your child interested in?

Do a little experiment: spend just one day observing what you talk about with your child, apart from daily needs like eating, dressing, clearing up or brushing teeth.

- What are the topics you talk about?
- What questions do they ask?
- What do you laugh about together?
- What was the last thing you discovered together?

Many parents can't think of any answers to these questions. Is this true of you?

Showing our own interest

Adults and children alike benefit when we can place more importance on the here and now. Try going for more walks together or walk where you have to go instead of driving. (In a car, the world flies by, making it difficult to explore or discover much.) Children want to ground themselves here in the world. Help them by going out on foot and looking at things through a child's eyes, as if they were completely fresh and new. Go on a voyage of discovery: What kind of tree is that outside the house? What is it called? And the one next to it? And what are the flowers? What kind of smell do they have?

'Is this really so important?' many may ask. I would argue that it is. We can only get to know and love the world, respect and protect it, by approaching it with interest.

Parents don't have to know all the answers

We should try to be authentic and admit, 'I don't know. Let's find out.' And then really go ahead and investigate.

We can prompt curiosity: 'What is actually in our breakfast muesli? Spelt flakes! Spelt – what's that? What does it look like? Where does it grow? And what else is in the muesli? Raisins, hazelnuts, milk. Where do they all come from? Let's find out!' Our enthusiasm can be infectious and help children become interested too. What helps everyone develop is the attitude that we can learn something new every day.

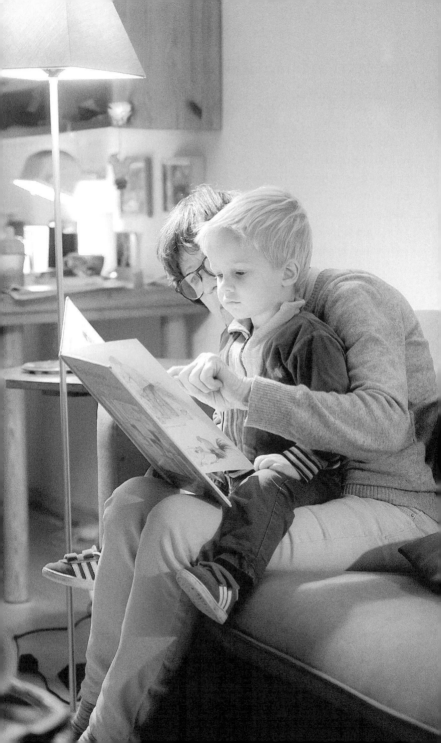

A Well-Nourished Soul

A mother is with her daughter in a supermarket, looking at the sweets. 'You can choose something,' she says. But the little girl doesn't. 'Come on, tell me what you'd like.'

Another shopper standing nearby says, 'Perhaps she wants something quite different...'

What the other shopper is trying to hint at is that of course children enjoy treats from time to time, but what they really need is not a treat or indeed any material gift. There are many children today who seem to get every object available but still lack something essential: nourishment for the soul.

What nourishes the soul?

When we meet our children one-to-one, it is very important to look them in the eyes. We can tell how much this contact means from the open-heartedness we feel in the interaction.

We can tell, too, when young children say 'Again!' When do they say this? When they hear lovely sounds that we sing, when we tell stories, when we play little rhyme games like 'Round and Round the Garden' or 'This Little Piggy went to Market'.

What happens in the gaze between Mum or Dad and children during these activities deeply touches both older and younger. This is precisely what creates the underlying warmth of soul that children need to thrive. Beautiful warm tones give wings to children's hearts and help them surmount all sorts of obstacles.

Take a look at this scene:

A father takes his two year old to the delivery ward to visit Mummy and the new baby. The young boy is standing there feeling a little lost. When his father sees this, instead of speaking to him rationally, he does what children long for if a situation feels uncomfortable: he starts to sing – as well as he can – a lovely children's song about dancing with your little brother. And at the same time he takes his child's hands and does a little dance with him.

The little boy looks radiant and cries out, 'Again!'

Singing together

Singing little songs and rhymes and playing games with our children is a simple pleasure. We can do it any time – when waiting, for instance. Notice something astonishing: when we begin to sing, our voices lift as if by themselves into a higher pitch, and this means that children are suddenly 'all ears'.

Try to reawaken childhood memories of old songs or rhymes, like 'Pat-a-cake, pat-a-cake baker's man', or 'Here is a church and here is a steeple…'

An alternative is to look up a few short nursery rhymes, write down the words and look at them beforehand. Very soon you'll come to know them by heart, as will your children, for children learn rhyming verses very quickly and easily.

Again!

I'm thinking of the face of a little girl who was so happy when her mother played a simple rhyming game with her. First the mother circled her finger on the girl's palm, then she finger-stepped up her arm to tickle her gently under the armpit.

Round and round the garden
like a teddy bear,
one step, two step
tickle under there!

Or up to her ear with this one:

Here's a little mouse
A wee little mouse,
Ding-a-ling-a-ling:
Is this your house?

'Again!' cried the child. And 'Again!' And once more: 'Again!'

This 'Again!', which comes from deep in a child's heart, is a sure sign they have found the soul food they need.

Sing a little song

Everything goes more smoothly if you sing along. Even clearing up after play can be fun if we start it off with a little tidying-up song:

Time to tidy up now
We've had a lovely play:
Let's tidy up together
Put everything away.

And since we, as parents, set an example to our children, we should of course be clearing away too, until children get the hang of it and know what to do. Sing a little song whenever it's time to tidy. We cannot sing too much!

Starting well is half the battle

In the morning, too, when it's time to get up, a cheerful song staves off moaning, grumpiness and having to pull blankets off reluctant young ones. Parents often reject this idea, saying, 'I'm grumpy myself in the morning, so singing doesn't come easily.' But give it a go sometime.

Try not to let self-consciousness get in the way of good feeling. Children won't ever judge our musical abilities. For them, singing is as natural and essential as breathing.

Singing nurtures mental development

Music researcher Andreas Mohr has discovered that 'without singing, especially in early childhood, specific neuronal networks are not, or are only imperfectly, established, leading to poorer brain function'.[14] So if we sing with our children it makes them more intelligent!

Singing to children also calms them swiftly if they are upset. Singing lowers the level of the stress hormone cortisol in the blood. Calming words are not quite as effective or as long-lasting.

Don't delegate childcare to a device

Bedtime rituals can send children off to sleep feeling nourished and loved, yet many parents leave this job to technology. 'Before she goes to bed I let my child watch her favourite programme,' one father told me at a parenting workshop. And a mother said, 'She listens to a story CD at the end of the day.'

It will not occur to young children to question why their parents trust a machine to help them prepare for bedtime, yet when we ourselves make the effort to be there for them, they will appreciate being sent off to sleep with the real nourishment of personal warmth.

Prayers

Many parents feel awkward about praying with children at bedtime or feel it is inappropriate as they have a secular home. But it is worth thinking about what prayer brings, and wondering how that richness can be brought into your family life, whatever your beliefs. As Albert Schweitzer says, the dire problem of our culture is that it has developed far further materially than spiritually.[15]

At the transition into the world of sleep, children are comforted by the idea that a higher world exists, a power that has made flowers, trees, animals, mountains, water, even stones and crystals.

Looking back on his own childhood, one father told me, 'I had the good fortune that my parents prayed with me.' When I asked why this was 'good fortune', he replied that he had never been afraid of night or the dark as a child. He put this down to his parents helping him go to sleep gently and creating a safe, nurturing atmosphere during prayers.

Children will sense intuitively whether an evening prayer is authentic for their parents; they will be able to tell whether they mean it. If this isn't something that's right for you, there are other ways of creating a wholesome, harmonious mood for sleep.

'What was lovely about today?'

Children love this question, as it gives a way of looking back together on the shared experience of the day.

'At bedtime we always light an evening candle,' one child told me. 'And then each person says what was lovely about the day. I like that very much, because there is always such a nice feeling.'

This kind of ritual can create a reassuring mood, which children need.

A parent told me, 'Each evening we used to sing "Twinkle, Twinkle Little Star" together, or say this poem by William Blake. The children still love it, even though they are eleven and twelve now.'

The sun descending in the west,
The evening star does shine;
The birds are silent in their nest,
And I must seek for mine.
The moon like a flower
In heaven's high bower,
With silent delight
Sits and smiles on the night.

Farewell green fields and happy grove,
Where flocks have took delight.
Where lambs have nibbled, silent move
The feet of angels bright;
Unseen they pour blessing
And joy without ceasing
On each bud and blossom
And each sleeping bosom.

Children's souls are also nourished if we play them soothing instrumental music or tell them a story or read them a fairy tale.

Starry Gold

One mother told me, 'I always sprinkle starry gold for my little ones.' I asked her what she meant, and she described her bedtime ritual every night. She tiptoes quietly to the window, reaches her hand out and then 'picks starry gold' to dust over each child, so that they have good dreams.

'But if it's cloudy, or raining?' I asked.

'The stars are still there always, even if you can't see them,' she replied with a smile.

How right she was. They are always there, like guardian angels. Children know this.

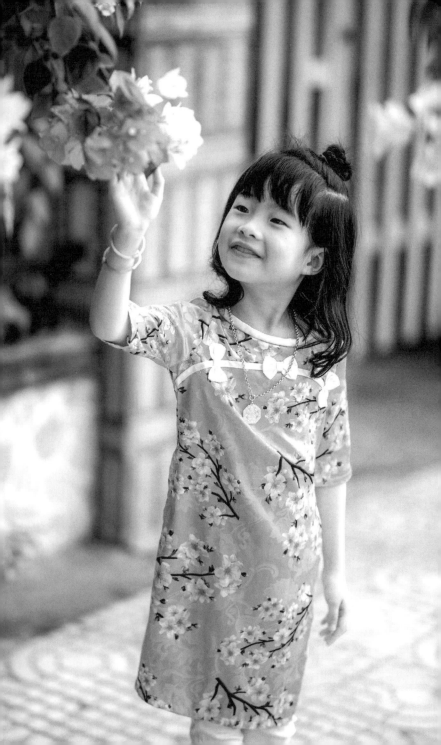

A Sense of Beauty

There are images and messages everywhere that we adults scarcely register, because we are so used to them. But infants see them: everything makes an impression on the very young.

A little boy and his father passed a big poster advertising a film. The image showed spurting blood.
'What's that?' the boy asked.
The father replied, 'It's ugly. I don't even want to look at it.'

It is certainly difficult to know what to do when a child asks a question like this. Should the father have stopped and explained or discussed the image? With an older child that would have been a good idea, but rational explanations carry little weight with a younger child who does not yet have the life experience to make sense of such images. Instead, as this father did, parents can simply take a clear stance and express it.

Everything we see has an effect, as Goethe knew:

Idiocy placed before our sight
Has a magical might:
When it claims our vision
Our spirit is imprisoned.[16]

Negative things, whether accidents, ugly objects or alarming images, have a magical power of attraction. They lure our gaze, as we all know.

It can be difficult to avoid these negative images. We even find skull motifs on young children's clothing nowadays.

One mother told me, 'My son went on at me for ages to buy him a skull jumper. He was even willing to break his piggy bank to help pay for it. And in the end I gave in and bought it for him.'

The mother in this example was trying to make her son happy by letting him have the jumper he wanted. However, if we feel uncomfortable with the things our children want, we can remember that wishes are not commands. If we stand up for our values as parents, our children will ultimately feel more secure.

Parents can say, 'That's ugly. I'm not buying it. I won't have something like that at home.' They may, through this, instil their values in their children, or at least give them pause for thought. Even if children do play with such 'fashionable' things somewhere else (say, at a friend's house) at home *you* can say what goes and what doesn't in your own family.

Developing an aesthetic sense

As parents, we can take the ugly and destructive motifs in visual culture as extra incentive to cultivate a sense of aesthetics in our children. Simple beauty enriches lives.

Toys are a good place to start. Children today usually have too many and the bedrooms of even very young children often look like toyshops. Some of the things may be lovely, but the overall impression is chaotic. Having too many objects in a room or on show impedes children's ability to play and can render them helpless before too many options.[17]

We can help by looking at our children's bedrooms and noticing what is really aesthetic or beautiful, and what we might quietly remove. What should we do with all the extra toys? Give them away, or store them in a cardboard box up in the loft and then occasionally swap them with the toys in the bedroom. They will feel like new toys to children who haven't seen them for a while.

Besides being expensive, the materials many toys are made of harm the environment. Toys made of natural materials such as wood are aesthetically pleasing and often better for stimulating the imagination. This is of key importance but often overlooked. Rudolf Steiner points out that 'the imagination works on the forms of the brain. The imagination develops the brain in the same way that the muscles of the hand are developed through corresponding work.'[18]

A beautiful dining table

Bringing beauty into everyday life helps children develop a sustaining sense of appreciation for small, ordinary blessings.

At dinnertime, for instance, try sitting down to a beautifully laid table without phones or other devices present. Meals are not just about preventing hunger. The dining table can become a shared, communal place of warmth and conviviality, a place where we really eat *together*. Eating at least once a day at a beautifully laid table feeds the eye as well as the stomach.

A beautiful table also encourages people, big or small, to eat in a calmer fashion. Consider this example:

A mother who had become tired of going on at her two boys about their table manners told me she'd found a new solution: 'For a while we've been playing the game "restaurant eating" at the weekend: we lay the table beautifully with a cloth, napkins, flowers and a candle. And it's amazing what an effect this has. We have lovely conversations, and I no longer have to keep hassling them about eating so messily. They don't!'

Ask children to help

Encourage children to help lay the table well from a young age. This will be two or three minutes of time very well spent. It will give pleasure to the children and the whole family. Praise children when they show care for how things look: 'You did that beautifully.'

And make sure nothing is missing before you sit down to eat. The aesthetic sense is enhanced if everyone can stay sitting at table and no one has to keep getting up to fetch something. It also lets you concentrate on your meal and on enjoying each other's company. 'We don't have the time,' many parents say. But beauty can be simple.

Beauty enhances understanding

It can be argued that a 'utilitarian' outlook disadvantages children. In his *Letters on the Aesthetic Education of Man*, Friedrich Schiller writes, 'There is no way to render our sense of nature comprehensible other than by first rendering it aesthetic.'[19] He means that our powers of reason depend on our aesthetic sense. However, we cannot rely on schools to instil an aesthetic sense in our children since aesthetic education is not covered in the internationally adopted PISA standards. This presents a valuable opportunity for us to cultivate it at home in daily life instead.

Everything has its place

We may have to work hard to create a sense that everything in our home has a rightful place. Try to clear up toys at the end of every day, preferably at the same time each evening. Don't expect your children to be able to do this straight away, but practise will help develop their sense of order. Take delight with children in the outcome, enjoy the pleasure gained from the labour: 'Look how neat and tidy the room is now.'

The other advantage of tidying up at the end of each day is that it becomes much easier to get children to bed. There is a calmer atmosphere because a tidy room tells them that the day is over.

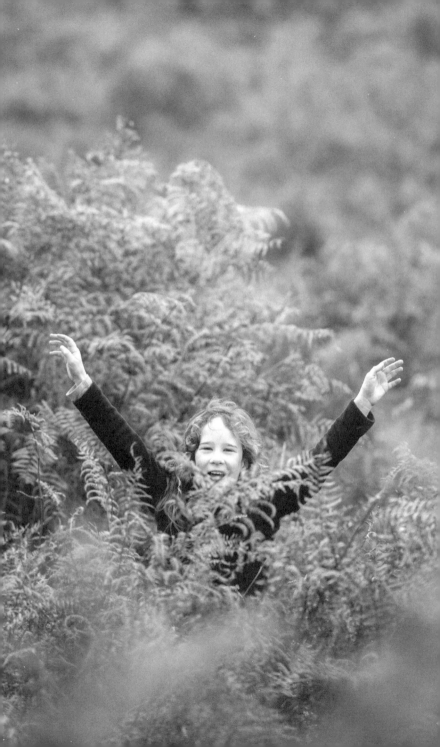

Connection with Nature

'My son can already download apps on my smartphone,' says the proud mother of a four year old. 'He likes playing farmyard games, and he learns a lot from them.'

The mother in this example might be proud of her son's accomplishments, but how much can children really learn about life from games on a screen? If we were to ask this boy what colour ducks are, he would probably say 'yellow'. Likewise, if we ask a group of children where milk comes from, they are likely to say 'the supermarket'. And eggs, honey or apples? The same. Nowadays it is common to see children tapping on a phone very fast, and they know lots of things – but not about the world immediately around them. If we ask them a couple of simple questions we'll often find they lack rapport with nature.

Children learn best through activity and motion, by being engaged with all their senses. They are indifferent to what they don't know at first hand, and they cannot value what they are indifferent to.

Living with the elements

Concrete, glass and technology are not child-friendly. The psychoanalyst Alexander Mitscherlich writes,

> A young person needs elemental things: water, mud, bushes, room to play. He can also come to awareness

amongst carpets, toy animals, and on tarmac roads and yards. He'll survive – but one shouldn't be surprised if he later fails to learn some basic social skills.[20]

Talking with parents suggests to me that this is true. One father described how he once pointed out a glorious evening sky to his ten-year-old son. Completely uninterested, the boy said, 'So what?' and turned his gaze back to his phone display.

Early engagement with nature

When children become familiar with the natural world from infancy, they don't suddenly get alarmed if they see an earwig. Children who hardly ever go out can perceive nature as frightening.

A boy has to go into the woods as part of a school project. Seeing some beetles, he cries out, 'Yuck, what are *those*?' He is alarmed because he doesn't have a spray to 'kill them all'.[21]

No parent wants their child to become this alienated from the real world, but this begs the question…

Do you let your child get dirty outdoors?

From talking to parents, I find the prevailing attitude is: 'We let our children play outside, as long as they don't get their clothes dirty.' Yet nature is not a clinical environment. A connection with nature comes about by direct contact, through all the senses, when children see, touch, smell, taste and feel earth, water, mud, sand, grass, trees and bushes. We should encourage them to play freely, climb trees, balance, run, hide, dig and build.

'You're dirty,' says a mother to her little daughter when she comes back from a walk with her dad. 'I'll have to put another load of washing on!'

The father replies, 'I just wanted her to feel free.'

It is not a matter of who is 'right' here but of what nurtures healthy development. Dirty clothes can be washed. Children thrive when they are allowed to play freely and intuitively in nature, when they learn to appreciate the way the earth feels and how to relate to its creatures.

How to cultivate a love of nature

I talk to two parents who take their children holidaying on a farm where they can help feed chickens, milk cows, muck out barns and bring the animals fresh hay. They tell of the pleasure their children have in stroking the young calves, how they laugh when one licks their hands all over with its long tongue. Each time they return home from these holidays, the parents say, the children's 'farm games' go on for weeks afterwards.

Not everybody has a garden or is able to holiday on a farm, but there are other opportunities to seek out nature. Is there a farm or market garden or an apiary in your neighbourhood? You could ask whether children can visit. There are also many urban gardening initiatives nowadays, and city farms, or allotments where families can rent a plot of land and try growing their own food.

Being out among growing things benefits children more than watching nature or farming films on TV, especially if they're allowed and encouraged to help. After a day's work and play outside they will go home feeling happy and fulfilled.

Nature on the windowsill

Direct experience is always the best way to get close to plants and growth, even if this is, to begin with, only on your windowsill. Sow cress seeds in a dish or saucer, water them carefully, and see how the seeds soon swell and germinate. After only a few days you can harvest and serve the fresh green seedlings. All kinds of seeds and grains can be planted in a flowerpot at home.

A father I know had a good idea after his children had eaten apples. 'If we plant the seeds,' he said, 'new apple trees will grow.'

The children were immediately enthusiastic and wanted to plant them right away.

'First of all we have to dry them,' he explained.

Having to wait a few days made things even more exciting. When the day for planting arrived, the children pushed the seeds deep into soil – nearly as deep as the length of a match. Then the pot was placed on the windowsill. 'Now we must water them every day, so they stay nice and moist,' said the father.

The children keep looking to see if anything was peeking out. And yes! One day it happened. A tiny seedling poked through the soil!

If you haven't ever witnessed it yourself, you might not believe how happy children are to watch something growing and developing. Give it a try.

Little children feel close to nature

Young children have no inherent fear of snails, spiders, ants or beetles. On the contrary, as long as no one prevents them ('Ugh, don't touch that!') they are interested in everything that is alive, everything that flies, crawls, scuttles and moves.

Children love to go out into nature, and there are so many fascinating things for young world-explorers to discover if they can roam freely in grass, sand and puddles, or amongst pine cones, sticks, stones, bushes, trees and leaves. Even an outing in a city park can be full of wonder:

'Walk! Walk!' cries a boy of about fifteen months when his mother takes him out in the buggy. Arriving at the park, at last he is allowed to run. He immediately starts investigating his surroundings, picking things up, touching everything and wondering. 'Look!' he calls, and brings his mother a small pebble. Then a leaf. And another. And then a stick.

She gladly receives the little treasures he brings her, and gives the child time to make his discoveries.

Close observation

Being a parent is a perfect opportunity to re-awaken the child inside us.

'Look,' said a girl in a group of children out on a walk. She pointed to a snail.

They all squatted down to see, and the parents joined them.

'Do you see its eyes?' her parents asked.

'Where?' she asked.

'Right at the end of the feelers. Those little dark points at the end.'

Very carefully the father moves his fingers close to the two upper feelers. And – hey presto – the snail withdraws them. Soon afterwards it carefully extends one and then the other feeler again. The children watch and wonder at this little miracle of nature.

Before they continue their walk, one of them places the snail very carefully in the grass beside the path so that 'it doesn't get run over by a bicycle'.

Such brief moments, with their close observation, awaken a real connection with nature and a sense of care for other creatures, however small.

Rejuvenation

Nature refreshes and rejuvenates us. When we are weary, it helps to go out into the open air, to a meadow or waterfall or a stream beneath trees. Or simply to go for a walk.

Walking barefoot is another wonderful way of connecting directly with nature. We can forget some of the thoughts that crowd our head by earthing ourselves to the sand or ground or grass with bare feet.

Climb a tree. Dam a brook. Splash.

Learning names for trees, flowers and birds

When children ask, 'What kind of tree is that?' perhaps not many of us know the answer. But this is easy to put right. Get hold of small field guides and take them along on walks. Then children can help identify trees, flowers and birds. Feel the tree's bark with them. Pick a leaf. 'Look, it's heart-shaped. I wonder what kind of tree has heart-shaped leaves?'

Some parents ask, 'But what's the point?' I tell them that to be at home in our surroundings, we need to know things and their names. Besides, identification can give rise to all kinds of conversations with our children as we sharpen our powers of observation together. 'What's the name of that flower over there? Look, it's still flowering in November!' Go exploring and discover what's out there.

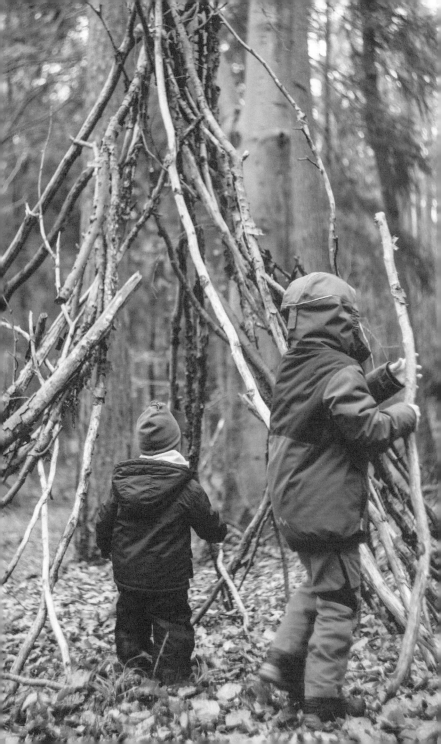

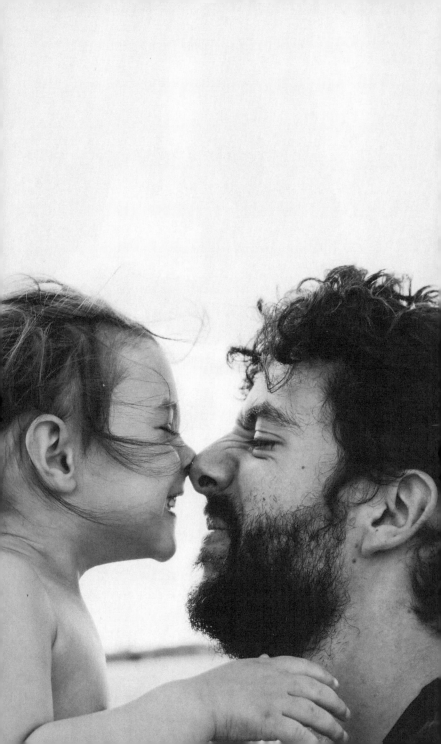

Humour and Light-Heartedness

Children love laughing

Children have a wonderful and infectious sense of humour. They love nothing better than lying on the floor, rolling with laughter. They also – often unintentionally – say funny things every day, so they will bring light-heartedness into adult life, if we look for it.

A four year old listened to the story of 'Mother Holle' and heard her described as having crooked teeth. He asked, 'Did she suck her thumb too?'

A parent told me, 'We were sitting together in a restaurant when the door opened and in came a man with a long, bushy beard. Our daughter called loudly, 'Look, it's a giant!'

Humour hamper

We all love to laugh with our children, and it's worth paying conscious attention to the things they say. It's easy to forget these conversations, so consider writing them down. Keep a journal and note each evening one moment of the day that made everyone smile or laugh. This is a lovely way of observing funny occurrences in daily family life, and over time it creates a 'humour hamper' from which to draw sustenance.

Meet mistakes with a light heart

Humour often flies out of the window when we feel we've done something wrong. Adults can take the lead on being more light-hearted when they make a mistake. Think about this example:

'I could kick myself,' says a father furiously. He has just burned the dinner while cooking. The whole family is immediately affected by his bad mood. There is cold bread and cheese for dinner, plus a large helping of stress and bad feeling for everyone.

Humour thrives best when it's clear that everyone makes mistakes sometimes. The famous clown Dimitri said, 'Laughter is healing.'[22]

We set a good example as parents if we can laugh at ourselves. Compare this example to the father with the burned dinner:

A father forgot a batch of biscuits and they burned. When he took the tray out of the oven he cried theatrically, 'Oh my goodness, they're all sootcrackers!'

Everyone laughed and the phrase entered their family history, so that from then on, they called anything that burned 'sootcrackers'!

Look at things from children's level

Children can really benefit when adults respond on their level.

A little boy who went to bed an hour before suddenly appeared in the living room again, saying 'I can't sleep! There's a lion under my bed.'

Instead of replying that this can't possibly be true, his father leapt up saying, 'Hang on, we'll sort that out!' He fetched a broom, swept vigorously under the bed and cried, 'Get out from under there, lion! Come on, I can see you! Go away, the door's over there!' He ran downstairs, flung the front door wide and shut it again with a bang. And then he came back to his son, saying, 'It's gone now. You can go to sleep.'

The child was amused, but also soothed and relieved by Daddy's warm-hearted action, and went peacefully to sleep.

Humour makes everything easier

'Did you wash your hands?' asks the father of a young girl.

'Ye-e-es,' says his daughter unconvincingly.

Her father raises one eyebrow and replies in a silly, mock-officious tone, 'I'm so terribly sorry, Madam, but I'm afraid it's just not going to be possible for me to believe that.'

The effect is instant: the girl goes off, giggling, and really does wash her hands this time.

Humour can achieve things much more easily than threats and anger – things like getting dressed, for instance.

A little boy is meant to put his shoes on, but refuses.

His mother calls, 'Let's see who'll be first, you or me,' lifts up her shoe and then pretends she is confused about where it goes and how to get it on.

The little boy meanwhile grabs his own shoes.

The mother opens her eyes wide in astonishment. 'What? You've already got one shoe on? I'd better hurry up.' She makes a show of clumsy speed.

The boy cries, 'I did it first!' and is terribly pleased.

They both laugh, and he helps his mother on with her second shoe.

Avoiding lectures

Humour can also come in handy in difficult situations with older children. As parents there is no need to discuss every decision with our children, nor do we need to justify ourselves if we have said we won't buy them something.

'I really need these new trainers,' a twelve year old demands.

'Ah,' his father replies with a wry smile. 'And what about a new hoodie? And new jeans? And a new phone, you must be *needing* that?'

The son rolls his eyes, but goes off without a murmur.

This father engages with his son, but his exaggeration shows without lecturing that the boy needs to revise his sense of the word 'need'!

Games keep us going

Play games with your children, especially ones with potential for mischief, such as hide-and-seek. Even older children love it if we pretend not to find one of them for ages, even though their hiding place is obvious.

Silly singing games can come in handy, for example when a child says they are too tired to walk any further.

A little boy's legs became weary when his family was out for a walk with a group of friends, and he was starting to complain. One of the grown-ups started singing, 'Noodle soup, noodle soup, everyone likes noodle soup!'

And then another parent sang, 'Lentil soup, lentil soup, everyone likes lentil soup!'

And the little one suddenly thought of another verse: 'Carrot soup...'

'I never knew how many different kinds of soup there were!' his mother said later. 'We thought of another and another, and then we were home!'

Wordplay and jokes

At school age, children laugh raucously at riddles, puns and wordplay, such as:

Why wouldn't the crab share his sweets?
Because he was a little shellfish.

What's faster, hot or cold?
Hot, because you can catch a cold.

Or knock-knock jokes:

Knock-knock.
Who's there?
A-tish
A-tish who?
Oh dear, I'm sorry, you sound like you've caught a cold!

Tongue-twisters are fun too, especially when they go wrong:

Red leather, yellow leather (repeated many times)

Peter Piper picked a peck of pickled peppers.
A peck of pickled peppers Peter Piper picked.
If Peter Piper picked a peck of pickled peppers,
Where's the peck of pickled peppers Peter Piper picked?
She sells seashells on the seashore.
The shells she sells are seashells, I'm sure.
For if she sells seashells on the seashore
Then I'm sure she sells seashore shells.

We can invent new ones with our children too.
And don't forget funny stories and tales. Read and laugh together.

Reversing roles

It's Saturday breakfast time. There's no rush or hurry today, so Dad decides to have some fun. He says to his children, 'You be the parents this morning, and we'll be the children.'

Role reversal is a very funny game to play with children over the age of five. Children usually portray adults very truthfully and it is highly amusing to see things from their point of view.

Here is a chance to know ourselves, laugh at ourselves and create family warmth and cheer.

Notes and References

1   Goethe, *Faust Part I,* Prelude
2   See the study [in German] on 'Motivation and Rewards'
    at http://www.sueddeutsche.de/wissen/motivation-und-
    belohnung-geld-macht-faul-1.156184
3   Alice Miller, *The Drama of the Gifted Child: The Search for the True
    Self,* Basic Books 2008.
4   Manfred Spitzer, *Vorsicht Bildschirm! Elektronische Medien,
    Gehirnentwicklung, Gesundheit und Gesellschaft,* Munich 2006.
5   In the interview 'Zu gut für das Kind', in the journal *Psychologie
    heute,* February 2010.
6   For more on these rules, see Christiane Kutik, *Stress-Free
    Parenting,* Floris Books, Edinburgh 2010, p. 18; and Christiane
    Kutik, *Entscheidende Kinderjahre,* Verlag Freies Geistesleben,
    Stuttgart 2012, p. 138.
7   See also Christiane Kutik, *Stress-Free Parenting,* op. cit,
    'Regeneration'.
8   For more on mirror neurones see Joachim Bauer,
    *Warum ich fühle, was du fühlst. Intuitive Kommunikation und das
    Gehimnis der Spiegelneurone,* Hamburg 2005.
9   Manfred Spitzer, *Vorsicht Bildschirm! Elektronische Medien,
    Gehirnentwicklung, Gesundheit und Gesellschaft,* Munich 2006.
10 See Rudolf Steiner, *Esoteric Development – Selected Lectures and
    Writings* (CW 245), Steiner Books 2003,
    Chapter 5, 'General requirements for Esoteric Development';
    Soul Exercises, CW 267, Steiner Books 2015; *Six Steps in Self-
    Development,* Rudolf Steiner Press 2010, page 38. Various
    authors have written about these exercises. See, for instance,
    Michael Lipson, *Stairway of Surprise. Six Steps to a Creative Life,*
    Anthroposophic Press 2002.

11 Jacob and Wilhelm Grimm, *An Illustrated Treasury of Grimm's Fairy Tales*, illustrated by Daniela Drescher, Floris Books, Edinburgh 2013; Jacob and Wilhelm Grimm, *A Favourite Collection of Grimm's Fairy Tales*, illustrated by Anastasiya Archipova, Floris Books, Edinburgh 2015.

12 From the poem by Reinhard Mey, 'Du bist ein Riese, Max', http://www.reinhard-mey.de/start/texte/alben/du-bist-ein-riese-max

13 Manfred Spitzer, *Digitale Demenz. Wie wir uns und unsere Kinder um den Verstand bringen,* Droemer Verlag, Munich 2014, p. 304.

14 Andreas Mohr, 5th Osnabrück Symposium, 'Singförderung im Kindesalter', see www.kinderstimmbildung.de

15 See *Das Buch der Albert Schweitzer Zitate*, Verlag C.H. Beck, Munich 2013, p. 94. From: Albert Schweitzer, *Kulturphilosophie I und II*, p. 90.

16 Johann Wolfgang Goethe, *Zahme Xenien.*

17 See Christiane Kutik, *Spielen macht Kinder stark*, Verlag Freies Geistesleben, Stuttgart 2013, the chapter 'Spielzeugflut.'

18 Rudolf Steiner, *Educating Children Today*, Rudolf Steiner Press 2008. GA 34 in the Complete Works.

19 Friedrich Schiller, *Letters Upon the Aesthetic Education of Man*, Kessinger Publishing 2004. See also the edition with commentary by Rudolf Steiner, and an introduction and afterword by Heinz Zimmermann, Verlag Freies Geistesleben, Stuttgart 2009, p. 132.

20 Alexander Mitscherlich, *Die Unwirtlichkeit unserer Städte,* Frankfurt am Main 1996 (special re-issue 2008).

21 Scene from the film *Play Again* at http://playagainfilm.com/

22 Clown Dimitri, *Humor: Gespräche über die Komik, das Lachen und den Narren*, with Corina Lanfranchi, Verlag am Goetheanum, Dornach 2000, p. 17.

Index

Stress-Free Parenting in 12 Steps

Christiane Kutik

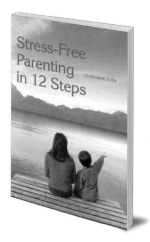

"If I had to choose just one book to give to a new parent, this one would be at the top of my list."
– *New View*

Written specifically for parents with no time and little energy, this concise, practical book highlights twelve simple steps for bringing some peace, composure and enjoyment back into everyday family life.

Also available as an eBook

florisbooks.co.uk

Parenting in the Here and Now

Realizing the Strengths You Already Have

Lea Page

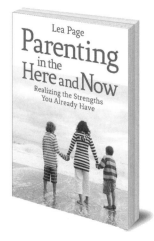

"An empowering guide to a truly heart-centered
way of parenting."
– Donna Simmons

Being a good parent doesn't mean being perfect, learning
complex theories or finding another twelve hours in the day.
Parenting in the Here and Now offers a refreshingly different
way. Rather than striving for – and failing to reach –
a frustrating ideal, parents can start from where they are
right now, and enjoy a more harmonious family life
almost immediately.

Also available as an eBook

florisbooks.co.uk

Warmth

Nurturing Children's Health and Wellbeing

Edmond Schoorel

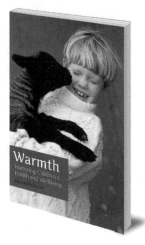

Warmth is one of the basic building blocks of existence; without it, there would be no life or growth. As parents we want our children to be warm – physically and emotionally.

In the first book of its kind, anthroposophical therapist Edmond Schoorel explores the role of warmth across many aspects of child development.

This fascinating and practical book gives parents and caregivers valuable insight into how to nurture different aspects warmth in everyday family life.

Also available as an eBook

florisbooks.co.uk